The Cancer Survivor's Handbook

TERRY PRIESTMAN is Consultant Clinical Oncologist working at New Cross Hospital, Wolverhampton. He is also Medical Reviewer for the charity Cancerbackup (which provides information for cancer patients, their relatives and health care professionals). He is a past Dean of the faculty of Clinical Oncology at the Royal College of Radiologists, and has written more than 100 papers in the medical press. He is also the author of *Coping with Chemotherapy* (2005), *Coping with Breast Cancer* (2006), *Coping with Radiotherapy* (2007) and *Reducing Your Risk of Cancer* (2008), all published by Sheldon Press.

Overcoming Common Problems Series

Selected titles

A full list of titles is available from Sheldon Press,
36 Causton Street, London SW1P 4ST and on our website at
www.sheldonpress.co.uk

The Assertiveness Handbook
Mary Hartley

Assertiveness: Step by step
Dr Windy Dryden and Daniel Constantinou

Body Language: What you need to know
David Cohen

Breaking Free
Carolyn Ainscough and Kay Toon

Calm Down
Paul Hauck

The Candida Diet Book
Karen Brody

Cataract: What you need to know
Mark Watts

The Chronic Fatigue Healing Diet
Christine Craggs-Hinton

The Chronic Pain Diet Book
Neville Shone

Cider Vinegar
Margaret Hills

The Complete Carer's Guide
Bridget McCall

The Confidence Book
Gordon Lamont

Confidence Works
Gladeana McMahon

Coping Successfully with Pain
Neville Shone

Coping Successfully with Panic Attacks
Shirley Trickett

Coping Successfully with Period Problems
Mary-Claire Mason

Coping Successfully with Psoriasis
Christine Craggs-Hinton

Coping Successfully with Ulcerative Colitis
Peter Cartwright

Coping Successfully with Varicose Veins
Christine Craggs-Hinton

Coping Successfully with Your Hiatus Hernia
Dr Tom Smith

Coping Successfully with Your Irritable Bowel
Rosemary Nicol

Coping with Age-related Memory Loss
Dr Tom Smith

Coping with Alopecia
Dr Nigel Hunt and Dr Sue McHale

Coping with Birth Trauma and Postnatal Depression
Lucy Jolin

Coping with Bowel Cancer
Dr Tom Smith

Coping with Brain Injury
Maggie Rich

Coping with Candida
Shirley Trickett

Coping with Chemotherapy
Dr Terry Priestman

Coping with Childhood Allergies
Jill Eckersley

Coping with Childhood Asthma
Jill Eckersley

Coping with Chronic Fatigue
Trudie Chalder

Coping with Coeliac Disease
Karen Brody

Coping with Compulsive Eating
Ruth Searle

Coping with Diabetes in Childhood and Adolescence
Dr Philippa Kaye

Coping with Diverticulitis
Peter Cartwright

Coping with Down's Syndrome
Fiona Marshall

Coping with Dyspraxia
Jill Eckersley

Overcoming Common Problems Series

Overcoming Common Problems Series

Living with Crohn's Disease
Dr Joan Gomez

Living with Eczema
Jill Eckersley

Living with Fibromyalgia
Christine Craggs-Hinton

Living with Food Intolerance
Alex Gazzola

Living with Grief
Dr Tony Lake

Living with Heart Failure
Susan Elliot-Wright

Living with Loss and Grief
Julia Tugendhat

Living with Lupus
Philippa Pigache

Living with Osteoarthritis
Dr Patricia Gilbert

Living with Osteoporosis
Dr Joan Gomez

Living with Rheumatoid Arthritis
Philippa Pigache

Living with Schizophrenia
Dr Neel Burton and Dr Phil Davison

Living with a Seriously Ill Child
Dr Jan Aldridge

Living with Sjögren's Syndrome
Sue Dyson

Losing a Baby
Sarah Ewing

Losing a Child
Linda Hurcombe

The Multiple Sclerosis Diet Book
Tessa Buckley

Osteoporosis: Prevent and treat
Dr Tom Smith

Overcoming Agoraphobia
Melissa Murphy

Overcoming Anorexia
Professor J. Hubert Lacey, Christine Craggs-Hinton and Kate Robinson

Overcoming Anxiety
Dr Windy Dryden

Overcoming Back Pain
Dr Tom Smith

Overcoming Depression
Dr Windy Dryden and Sarah Opie

Overcoming Emotional Abuse
Susan Elliot-Wright

Overcoming Hurt
Dr Windy Dryden

Overcoming Insomnia
Susan Elliot-Wright

Overcoming Jealousy
Dr Windy Dryden

Overcoming Procrastination
Dr Windy Dryden

Overcoming Shyness and Social Anxiety
Ruth Searle

Overcoming Tiredness and Exhaustion
Fiona Marshall

The PMS Handbook
Theresa Cheung

Reducing Your Risk of Cancer
Dr Terry Priestman

Safe Dieting for Teens
Linda Ojeda

The Self-Esteem Journal
Alison Waines

Simplify Your Life
Naomi Saunders

Stammering: Advice for all ages
Renée Byrne and Louise Wright

Stress-related Illness
Dr Tim Cantopher

Ten Steps to Positive Living
Dr Windy Dryden

Think Your Way to Happiness
Dr Windy Dryden and Jack Gordon

The Thinking Person's Guide to Happiness
Ruth Searle

Tranquillizers and Antidepressants: When to start them, how to stop
Professor Malcolm Lader

The Traveller's Good Health Guide
Dr Ted Lankester

Treating Arthritis Diet Book
Margaret Hills

Treating Arthritis: The drug-free way
Margaret Hills

Treating Arthritis: More drug-free ways
Margaret Hills

Understanding Obsessions and Compulsions
Dr Frank Tallis

When Someone You Love Has Depression
Barbara Baker

Overcoming Common Problems

The Cancer Survivor's Handbook

DR TERRY PRIESTMAN

sheldon PRESS

First published in Great Britain in 2009

Sheldon Press
36 Causton Street
London SW1P 4ST

The author and publisher have made every effort to ensure that the
external website and email addresses included in this book are correct and
up to date at the time of going to press. The author and publisher are not
responsible for the content, quality or continuing accessibility of the sites.

British Library Cataloguing-in-Publication Data
A catalogue record for this book is available from the British Library

ISBN 978–1–84709–048–5

1 3 5 7 9 10 8 6 4 2

Typeset by Fakenham Photosetting Ltd, Fakenham, Norfolk
Printed in Great Britain by Ashford Colour Press

Produced on paper from sustainable forests

Contents

Note to the reader

This is not a medical book and is not intended to replace advice from your doctor. Consult your pharmacist or doctor if you believe you have any of the symptoms described, and if you think you might need medical help.

Introduction

When I first started working in cancer treatment the first question almost everybody asked me when they discovered what I did was 'Will they ever find a cure?' That was 40 years ago. What amazes me is that I still get asked the same question today. During the past four decades progress in cancer treatment has been amazing. The outlook in many different types of cancer has been transformed, such that now more than half of all people diagnosed with cancer in the UK can expect to be cured, and of those who can't be permanently cured, many will have years of virtually normal life, after their treatment, before their disease reappears.

Successes in the field of oncology since the 1960s have been remarkable and have been achieved by the discovery of new treatments, and their introduction after rigorous clinical trials proving their worth. However, one consequence of all this success has, until very recently, been virtually overlooked by health care professionals: the fact that more and more people will be long-term survivors, with a normal life expectancy, after their cancer treatment. The focus has always been on improving treatments and increasing cure rates, and what happens to people after that has largely been ignored – if you're cured, surely that's all that matters.

The picture is changing, however, and there is increasing realization that life after cancer may not be as simple as all that. For some people cancer may be a life changing experience in a positive way; it may give them a new appreciation of life and allow them to savour every extra minute, or it may offer them the opportunity for a new beginning, having been spiritually strengthened by the cancer journey, to find a fresh vision of what life is all about. All too often there are problems as well, however, and the fact that life has changed dramatically may have its negative side.

Studies in the USA have highlighted problems, and in the UK the Government's 2007 Cancer Reform Strategy document, setting out the agenda for the next decade, had a whole section devoted to the issue of 'Cancer survivorship' and outlined a new 'National Cancer Survivorship Initiative', which the Department of Health was to take forward in partnership with Macmillan Cancer Support and other cancer charities. So the tide is turning, and the needs of people who survive cancer are beginning to be understood.

This book is intended as a step along that road, providing a simple explanation of some of the issues that people living after cancer might face and, I hope, giving some bits of helpful advice. The book is divided very roughly into two halves: the first deals with medical aspects, and the second covers issues related to everyday life. This is a new area, and it is still one aspect of cancer in which relatively little research has been done and relatively little has been written, but – with any luck – that is about to change.

Terry Priestman

1

Am I cured?

You have reached the end of your treatment. That treatment may have involved major surgery, weeks of radiotherapy, months of chemotherapy and possibly years of hormone therapy. Throughout that time, one of the things that will have kept you going was the hope or the expectation that once it was all over you would be cured – the cancer would be gone, never to return. So, you see your specialist and you ask that all important question: 'Has it worked, am I cured, has the cancer gone for good?'

Unfortunately, there is no way to know for certain. The best your doctor can do is give you an idea of how likely it is that all will be well, but there is no way that they can give you a guarantee that everything will be all right. They may be pretty sure that your cancer has gone, but they can never be absolutely certain. Why not? Surely they are the experts, with years of experience and training, and the back up of amazingly sophisticated technology: CT scans, MRI scans, PET scans and a galaxy of blood tests and other investigations. With all that expertise and all those resources, surely they must have the answer.

How cancers grow

To understand their difficulty, we need to look at a bit of basic cancer biology. Back in the 1960s a scientist in the USA, Howard Skipper, conducted an experiment in which he injected a single leukaemic blood cell into a mouse whose immune system had been suppressed, so that it could not reject the cell. A couple of weeks later the mouse was dead from acute leukaemia. This

1

showed that a fatal cancer could develop from changes in just a single cell; all it needed was for a genetic change, a mutation, to take place in a solitary cell among all of the billions in our bodies for a potentially lethal cancer to be triggered.

Once that first cancer cell develops, it will divide and multiply; the one cell will become two, the two will become four, the four will become eight, and so on. Tumour biologists call each of these multiplications a 'doubling', which is logical enough because each time they happen the number of cancer cells is doubled. After about 20 doublings that solitary cancer cell will have become a mass of one thousand million (10^9) cancer cells. That sounds an awful lot, but in fact it amounts to a lump no more than half a centimetre across, which is not quite the size of a baked bean.

However, this lump of 10^9 cancer cells, this mini baked bean sized tumour, is about the earliest stage that most cancers are likely to be discovered. A routine physical examination by a doctor, or a test like a scan or x-ray, is very unlikely to pick up anything much smaller than this. This means that it is possible to have tiny, microscopic seedlings of cancer in the body, which may contain tens or even hundreds of millions of cells, but which will still be completely undetectable. The only way of finding them would be to chop us up into tiny pieces and look at each bit under the microscope – not a very practical option.

Most cancers develop at a single site, in a single organ: a breast cancer in the breast, a prostate cancer in the prostate gland, a bowel cancer in the colon or the rectum, and so on. These are called primary cancers, the starting point for the disease. If these cancers are not treated they have the potential to spread, sending off minute clusters of cancer cells into the lymph system, to nearby lymph nodes or into the blood stream, and then to spread throughout the body to other organs such as the liver, the lungs or the bones. If no treatment is offered, these microscopic clusters will grow into secondary cancers, which are colonies of cells that have spread from the primary cancer to other parts of the body. These secondary cancers are also called metastases, so a primary cancer that has spread and given rise to secondary cancers is also called a metastatic cancer.

Armed with these basic facts about cancer growth, we can go back to our original problem of knowing whether treatment has brought about a cure. Let us take a specific example to explain this. A woman has a lump in her breast, tests show it is a cancer and there is no sign of any spread of the cancer elsewhere. She has surgery, to remove the primary tumour, followed by radiotherapy to the remaining breast tissue; as a precaution she also has six months of chemotherapy. At the end of that time a careful physical examination, and some routine tests, show no trace of any cancer. Is she cured? She may well be, but we can't be sure. It is just possible that before her primary cancer was removed it had sent off microscopic seedlings that could form secondary cancers. The hope is that if this had happened, then these tiny colonies would have been wiped out by the chemotherapy, but we can't be certain. Why is this? The answer is that even before we started any treatment there was no obvious sign of spread of her cancer, so if there were secondary tumours they had to be microscopic, undetectable. We could not say for sure whether they were there or not, and because we could not be sure whether they existed before treatment began, we have no way of telling whether they have gone, now that the treatment is finished. As far as we can tell, everything is clear, but we can't tell down to the last few tens or hundreds of millions of cancer cells. There could still be minute traces of the disease lurking somewhere in her body that could cause a problem in the years to come. We may be pretty sure that everything will be all right, but we can't be absolutely certain.

This may all sound rather negative. However, coming back to that fundamental question 'Am I cured?', although your specialist won't be able to give you a guarantee, what they can do is give you a very good idea of your chances of a cure, what the odds are that your treatment has been successful. They should be able to tell you whether the likelihood of your cancer coming back is very remote (a one in a hundred chance or less) or whether the risk is greater. How do they do this, how do they know what your chances are?

Calculating the odds

Many different factors affect the chances of a particular type of cancer being cured after treatment, and it is impossible to discuss all of these, but among the more important of these factors are the type of cancer, the stage of the cancer, the grade of cancer and the general health of the person who has the cancer.

The type of cancer

Cancer isn't a single disease. There are hundreds of different types of cancer. The likelihood of a permanent cure varies enormously between the different types. For example, about 96 out of 100 men with testicular cancer can expect to be cured whereas, at the other extreme, sadly only about two out of 100 people who develop a cancer of their pancreas are likely to survive for five years or more.

Stage

Even for a particular type of cancer there are huge variations in outcome, and a key factor here is the stage of the disease when it is first discovered. The stage of the cancer is a measure of how far it has progressed, how advanced or widespread the disease is. Doctors have devised systems for staging cancers that vary from cancer to cancer. Most of these are based on something called the 'TNM' system. In this system, 'T' describes the size and extent of the primary cancer, 'N' tells you whether the cancer has spread to nearby lymph nodes and 'M' indicates whether it has spread through the blood stream to other parts of the body. Although the TNM system provides a lot of detailed information about a cancer, it can be quite complicated and sometimes simpler systems are used instead. One of these is the Dukes staging system for bowel cancer, devised in the 1930s by a London pathologist called Cuthbert Dukes. We can use this as an example of how staging systems work. Dukes defined four stages of the disease.

- Stage A: the cancer only affects the lining of the wall of the bowel.
- Stage B: the cancer has eaten through the inner lining of the bowel into muscle coat of the bowel wall.
- Stage C: the cancer has spread into nearby lymph nodes.
- Stage D: the cancer has spread more distantly to form secondary cancers in the liver or the lungs.

The importance of these stages can be seen when we look at statistics for the chances of a cure. More than eight out of ten people with a bowel cancer that is stage A when it is first diagnosed will be cured; for those with stage B the figure falls to about six in ten; for stage C it is about four out of ten; and for stage D it drops to only about one in 20.

This pattern with bowel cancer is the same with all other types of cancer. The earlier the stage of the disease at the time when the cancer is first discovered, the more likely it is to be cured.

Once a cancer has been diagnosed, what usually happens next is that doctors conduct tests to try to find exactly what stage the cancer is. Once this is known it will guide their decisions about what treatment is best, and it will also give them some idea of the chances of that treatment being successful.

Grade

As well as knowing the stage of a cancer, knowing its 'grade' is also often very important. The grade of the cancer is worked out by looking at the appearance of the cancer cells under the microscope. Once again there is a number of grading systems in use for different cancers, but most rely on just three categories: grade I, grade II and grade III. In a grade I cancer the tumour cells look very much like the normal cells in the organ where the cancer has started; for example, in a grade I primary breast cancer the cancer cells will be very similar in appearance to the surrounding normal breast cells. In a grade III cancer the tumour cells look very abnormal and do not resemble the surrounding normal cells at all; they are obviously cancerous. In a grade II cancer the appearance of the cells is somewhere in between. There is a bit of medical jargon that goes with this, with grade I cancers being known as 'well differentiated', grade II cancers 'moderately differentiated' and Grade III cancers 'poorly differentiated'.

In general terms, grade III cancers tend to be more aggressive and more difficult to cure than grade II tumours, and grade I cancers tend to be less aggressive and more curable.

Health and fitness

A final factor to mention is the person's level of fitness and general health – whether he or she has other illnesses besides the cancer. As a rule, the healthier someone is at the time when the cancer is diagnosed, the better are the chances of a cure. This is in part because the person's immune system is likely to be better able to help them fight the disease, and their bodily fitness will increase their ability to cope with any side effects of treatment. Once again, doctors may use any of a variety of scales to score general wellbeing; one of the most widely used of these is the World Health Organization (WHO) performance score. This is graded 0 to 4 as follows.

0 You are fully active and more or less as you were before your illness.

1 You can't carry out heavy physical work but can do anything else.

2 You are up and about for more than half of the day; you can look after yourself but are not well enough to work.

3 You are in bed or sitting in a chair for more than half the day; you need some help to look after yourself.

4 You are in bed or a chair all of the time and need a lot of looking after.

Once your specialist knows the type of cancer you have, the stage and grade of your cancer, and has assessed your general fitness, then he or she can give you an idea of the chances that treatment will lead to a long-term cure. Specialists do this based on knowledge of the national statistics for outcomes of cancer treatment, which are collected by Cancer Registries across the country. So, for example, if you are a woman with an early stage malignant melanoma of the skin that has not spread to the lymph nodes or to other parts of your body, you have a grade I cancer and your WHO score is 0, then you have an almost 90 per cent chance of a cure. On the other hand, if you are someone with a lung cancer that has spread widely through your body, the tumour is grade III and your WHO score is 3, then sadly your chance of a cure is very poor; indeed, you would probably be too ill to read this book.

Beware of anecdotal evidence

These statistics are still only a guide, and they cannot tell for certain what will happen. As with bookmakers, who can give you the odds but can't guarantee who will win the race, these figures will give you an idea of your chances of a cure but they can't tell absolutely what will happen in your particular case. Having said this, they are the best guide we have at the moment and they are much more reliable than personal anecdotes. What I mean by this is that when many people first learn that they have cancer, their thoughts and feelings are coloured by what they have seen happen to friends and relatives who have been diagnosed with the disease in the past. Those experiences can often be very misleading. Just because, say, you had a grandmother who died from breast cancer, this does not mean that breast cancer can't be cured. Today, more than three out of every four women with breast cancer will be cured. Likewise, having had a young friend with Hodgkin's lymphoma who died of cancer does not mean that you will die if you get the disease; again, current figures show that more than eight out of ten people will be cured.

National statistics may not be a foolproof guide to what will happen to you, but they are a much better predictor than knowledge based on the experiences of a handful of acquaintances. Looking at what has happened to just a small number of individuals you know, or have heard about, and thinking that your experience will be the same as theirs, can be very misleading. National statistics may seem impersonal but they give a far more accurate picture of what your chances of success will be than relying on anecdotal evidence.

What does cure mean?

When someone who has had cancer asks his or her doctor if they have been cured, what they want to know is whether the treatment has permanently eliminated the cancer, so that it will never return and cause problems. However confident the medical team may be about the chances of success, they can never be 100 per cent sure that their treatment will have worked. Even with the most curable of cancers, there will still be the one person in a 1000 or even 10,000 in whom, for some reason, things do not work out as expected. The two main reasons for this uncertainty are doubts about whether the primary cancer has been completely removed, or destroyed, and whether there are any microscopic, invisible, secondary cancers that will continue to grow and cause problems in the future.

When a surgeon does an operation to remove a primary tumour, or when a clinical oncologist gives a course of radiotherapy to destroy a cancer, there is always the possibility – albeit usually a very slight one – that a few cancer cells may be missed and remain behind. Over time, which may be anything up to a year or two, these minute traces of tumour will grow and the cancer will reappear. When this happens, doctors call it a 'local recurrence' – the cancer reappearing in the same place as the original primary cancer.

The microscopic secondary cancers are tiny seedlings that have escaped into the blood stream or the lymphatic system some time before the primary cancer was treated (see page 2). If doctors feel that there is a strong risk that such seedlings might be present, they may provide extra treatments such as chemotherapy or hormone therapy to try and destroy them; this is called 'adjuvant treatment'. Adjuvant treatment is the treatment of a risk, not a certainty, and is given when doctors feel that the features of the primary cancer (such as its stage or grade) suggest that microscopic seedlings may have spread elsewhere, even though they are too small to be detectable. However, because these tiny secondary cancers are too small to be seen by the naked eye, or picked up by scans or x-rays, it is impossible to know for certain whether the adjuvant treatment will have got rid of them completely. If it hasn't, then over time – which once again may be a matter of some years, depending on the growth rate of the individual cancer – secondary cancers or metastases will finally appear and cause symptoms and problems.

Because there is always a risk that a local recurrence, or distant metastases, could appear at a later date, even if that risk is incredibly small, the only way that doctors can be really sure someone is completely cured is if, after a period of time, they are alive and well with no sign of their cancer having come back. Different types of cancer have very different rates of growth, and so the length of time you have to wait to be certain that you have the 'all clear' depends on the nature of your initial cancer.

When researchers first started looking at this question, in the 1930s, they studied people who had cancers of their mouth or throat (often called head and neck cancers). They discovered that if someone was alive, with no sign of local recurrence or distant metastases from one of these cancers, five years after their initial treatment, then the cancer never came back – they were cured. These early results led to the belief that if someone was well five years after cancer treatment, then they were cured. As time went on, however, it became clear that some types of cancer could still reappear, as either local recurrences or distant secondary cancers, more than five years after treatment of the primary cancer.

Medical statisticians puzzled over this and finally came up with an answer, which is a bit complicated and needs some explanation. What they did was study large numbers of people who had treatment for particular types of cancer and then followed them up for many years, seeing how many were alive and free from cancer each year. They compared these groups with a similar number of people, of similar age, from the 'normal' population. They then looked at the survival curves for each of the groups. Each year some people in the 'normal' group would die, from causes such as heart attacks, strokes or accidents. Similar numbers of people in the 'cancer' group would die of these causes, but there would also be some additional deaths caused by the cancer coming back. This meant that for some years the 'cancer' survival curve would fall more quickly than the 'normal' survival curve. After some years, however, no extra cancer deaths would occur, and the two survival curves would then become parallel. When this point was reached, with no more cancers coming back, you could then say that there was a cure.

These studies showed that for different types of cancer the time you had to wait after treatment of the primary cancer before you could be sure that there was a cure varied from five years to more than 20, although for most cancer types it was between five and ten years. What these findings also showed us was that most of the cancers that came back did so sooner rather than later, during the first two or three years after treatment. As time went by, and the closer it became to the time when you could say that particular type of cancer was cured, the fewer cancer related deaths there were.

Second cancers

One point that can be confusing is the difference between a cancer coming back and development of a new cancer. If someone has had a cancer treated, this doesn't mean that they will never get another cancer in the future. For example, a woman who has had a cancer of her cervix that was successfully treated when she was in her thirties could still develop a breast cancer when she was in her sixties, or a man who had curative treatment for a testicular cancer in his twenties might still get prostate cancer in his seventies. These people would be unlucky, but having had one cancer doesn't protect you from getting another.

Doctors call these new tumours 'second cancers'. These are different from 'secondary cancers', which are seedlings of tumour that have spread to other parts of the body from an original primary cancer.

Usually, having had a cancer doesn't put you at greater risk of developing another cancer, but there are exceptions to this. For instance, a heavy smoker who develops lung cancer and has this successfully treated is still at risk of developing other smoking-related cancers, such as bladder cancer or throat cancer, or even another lung cancer. If doctors feel that you have an increased chance of getting a second cancer, they will usually make sure you have regular check ups to look out for this and pick it up at its earliest, most curable stage.

So, when it comes to the question of 'a cure', where does all this clinical uncertainty and statistical complexity leave us? Well, although there are still no absolute guarantees, what we can say is that if you have no sign of your cancer having come back, or spread to other places, five years after your treatment ended then you are very likely to be cured, and if the same is true at ten years then you are almost certainly cured.

Other words doctors may use to describe the results of your treatment

A cure is the ultimate goal of cancer treatment, and happily today it is more often achieved than not. However, doctors use a number of other words and phrases to explain the results of therapy, and these different medical terms can be quite confusing. It is therefore worth spending a bit of time to try to understand some of them.

Remission and response

'Remission' and 'response' are very commonly used words and they mean the same: things are getting better as a result of treatment. Remissions/responses may be either partial or complete. A partial response means that the cancer has become smaller, but it has not disappeared. The exact definition of a partial response/remission varies. Over the years studies have shown that it is very difficult to measure small changes in a tumour's size accurately. Because of this, most clinical trials state that a cancer must shrink by 50 per cent or more before you can call it a partial response/remission. Even this is not straightforward, however, because some trials consider a halving in the diameter of a cancer to be a partial response/remission, whereas others look for a halving of its volume, and these definitions are very different. For instance, a 50 per cent reduction in diameter means that the tumour has shrunk much more than 50 per cent in volume. To make matters even more confusing, some specialists will state that if a cancer has reduced by 30 per cent, or even only 25 per cent, it can still be regarded a partial response/remission. As if this wasn't enough, experts also often introduce a time factor into their definition, saying that you can only call it a remission/response if it lasts for more than three months, whereas others require a minimum of one month and yet others think six months is the right figure! At the end of the day, keeping things simple, what a partial response/remission basically means is that the cancer has become noticeably smaller but hasn't disappeared.

In some ways, defining a complete response, or remission, is a bit easier; it is when all signs of the cancer have disappeared. This means that when your oncologist examines you, he or she can find no sign of the cancer, and any x-rays, scans or blood tests are completely clear. At first sight, it perhaps seems that this means that the cancer has been cured, but this may not be the case. Bear in mind that, as described above, there could still be microscopic traces of cancer, tiny seedlings of clusters of cancer cells, which are too small to show up on any physical examination or test (see page 2); over time these will carry on growing and eventually the cancer will return. Because of what they know about the way in which particular cancers respond to treatment, oncologists will usually have a good idea as to whether a complete response is likely to be temporary – lasting for anywhere from a few weeks to several years – or whether there is a good chance of a long-term cure. Unfortunately, as we have already seen, time is the only sure way to know that you have been cured. Achieving a complete response is an essential first step down that road.

Relapse

'Relapse' is the other side of the coin to remission and response; it means that the cancer has come back, or is getting larger rather than smaller – things are getting worse, not better. When someone has had treatment for a primary cancer, it may relapse either by coming back in the same place (a local recurrence) or by spreading to other places (secondary cancer or metastatic disease). To give an example, suppose a fit 70-year-old man develops a cancer in his prostate gland. Tests show that his cancer appears to be confined to his prostate and he decides to have a course of radiotherapy and some hormone treatment to get rid of it. At the end of his treatment, when the tests are repeated, there is no evidence of any cancer. He may well be cured, but if the cancer does come back – if he relapses – then this may be because it reappears in the prostate gland itself (a local recurrence) or because it has spread through the blood stream to one or more of the bones forming secondary cancers, or metastases, in one or more parts of the skeleton. Sometimes, the appearance of secondary cancers is called a 'distant' relapse, to distinguish it from a 'local' relapse.

When someone is having a cancer treated and achieves a partial response, with the tumour(s) having become smaller but not having disappeared, then he or she is said to have relapsed when the cancer begins to grow again – when it is getting bigger, not smaller. Once again, the exact definitions of 'relapse' in this situation are variable. Some people say the cancer(s) must grow by more than 25 per cent in size, whereas others use different measures. An alternative word used for this is 'progression'. So, with either relapse or progression of the cancer, the news is not good – things are getting worse, not better.

Stable disease and control

Sometimes someone may have a cancer that is not getting any bigger but is not getting any smaller either. Nothing much is changing. In this situation, the disease is said to be stable, or controlled. So if someone is told that his or her cancer is controlled, or stable, then it means that things aren't getting any better but they aren't getting any worse. With some types of cancer it may not be possible to get rid of them, or even to achieve remission with significant shrinkage of the tumour, but they can be controlled, or kept stable, often for long periods of time, perhaps many months or even years, allowing life to continue relatively normally.

Even if a cancer comes back, as a local recurrence or with distant secondaries, and the doctors say that it cannot be cured, further treatment can often bring about one or more remissions, and periods of stabilization, which can mean years of everyday life during which there may be very little in the way of symptoms and problems.

Survival

The way that doctors talk about 'survival' after a diagnosis of cancer can be very puzzling. They may talk about disease-free or relapse-free survival, or they may use the phrase overall survival. Disease-free survival and relapse-free survival mean the same: the length of time between someone having his or her cancer treated and that cancer coming back, as either a local recurrence or distant secondaries. Overall survival means the time from when the cancer is first treated to the time of death. An example might help to make this clearer. Suppose a 60-year-old man has an operation to remove a lung cancer. He is well for a while but six months later he develops secondary lung cancer in his liver. His relapse-free or disease-free survival has been six months. However, he then goes on to have chemotherapy, which gives him a remission, and when he relapses again he has some radiotherapy, which helps to control his disease, so he actually lives another 18 months after his cancer came back. So, his overall survival is two years: the six months from the time of treatment until he relapsed, plus the 18 months until he finally succumbs to his disease.

Many of the reports of clinical trials in cancer, published in medical journals, focus on the relapse-free survival times rather than overall survival. This is because one usually has to wait much longer, often many years, to know the overall survival figures for a group of patients, whereas reliable relapse-free numbers can be collected much sooner. Many experts argue that relapse-free survival figures are a good predictor of overall survival, but this is not always the case, so other experts feel that clinical trial results based on relapse-free survival data should be treated with some caution.

2

Follow up

When you have finished your treatment your hospital medical team will arrange for you to come and see them from time to time for a check up – 'follow up'. How often follow-up visits are booked, whom you see and what actually happens at these visits varies with different types of cancer, and also differs from hospital to hospital. There are very few guidelines about how follow up should be organized, and the pattern is extremely variable.

If you have a treatment for a simple skin cancer (a rodent ulcer or basal cell carcinoma), then you may only need one visit a few weeks later. For most cancers, however, follow up will go on for a number of years; five years is typical but for some tumours a much longer time will be needed. If all is well, then the interval between visits usually gets longer as time goes by; a typical pattern would be appointments every three months for the first year, every four months for the second year, then six monthly up to five years and annually thereafter.

Traditionally, follow-up checks are done by a doctor, but in some centres specialist nurses are now covering some of these duties. If your treatment involved several different consultants, for example if you had surgery, chemotherapy and radiotherapy, then you may find that you are given appointments for each of the three different medical teams, or your doctors may have agreed a system where just one of them looks after you. It is also very often the case that although your consultant(s) will make most of the decisions while you are having your treatment, and you will usually see quite a lot of him or her during this time, follow up visits are frequently in the hands of more junior members of the medical team; indeed, it is by no means rare for a person never to see the consultant again after their treatment is over.

At the present time there is also debate opening up about the role of family doctors, and their practice nurses, in the follow up of people who have had cancer. In the past this has been done exclusively by hospital teams, but many general practitioners (GPs) are arguing that they could do it just as well, and often more conveniently for the person, avoiding lengthy journeys to hospital. As a result of this, various studies are now underway to explore how GPs could play a greater part in the follow up process. Ideally, you should have a say in who does your follow up, but this is not always the case. If you do have any concerns, then do raise them with your medical team.

What happens at a follow-up visit

Follow-up visits will always involve some questions to find out how you are feeling, and there will usually be a physical examination as well. Whether any tests or investigations are needed is very variable, depending once again on your tumour type and on the preferences of individual specialists. If you have any new symptoms or problems, then these will always be investigated as needed. The role of routine tests for someone who is well with no obvious evidence of the cancer coming back is more complex, and controversial. In some cancers, for example breast cancer, extensive research has shown that if you have no symptoms, then special tests, such as scans and blood tests, will almost always be normal and there is no benefit in doing them. If you are not aware of a problem, then tests are very unlikely to find any evidence of your cancer coming back (the one test that is used routinely in breast cancer follow up is a regular mammogram, but the aim here is to detect possible second cancers that might have developed – new cancers – not to look for signs of your original cancer coming back). In contrast, in other cancers – testicular cancer is a good example – tests can pick up recurrent cancer at a very early stage, well before any symptoms appear, and so blood tests and scans are a routine part of the follow-up process.

A difficult aspect of routine testing is where the test may be able to detect a recurrence of the cancer before there are any symptoms, but there are no treatments available that will be able to cure that recurrence. Doctors differ in their approach here. Some do regular tests so they detect a recurrence as soon as possible, and then offer treatment that may help to control the disease even though it cannot cure it. Others wait until symptoms appear and then do tests to confirm that there is a recurrence, and then offer treatment to try to control it. There is no evidence that people live any longer with either one approach or the other. Looking at this from the patient's view-point, having routine tests means that many people get a lot of reassurance from knowing that those tests are normal. However, if one of your tests comes back abnormal, and an incurable recurrence is confirmed, then you will have the anxiety and stress of knowing that you have incurable cancer for far longer than someone who did not have the tests, and waited until they developed symptoms before the recurrence was diagnosed. If it made no difference to the actual length of life you had left, would you prefer to know that you had an incurable cancer sooner or later? I may be wrong, but I think that most doctors don't discuss this with their patients and tend to make the deci-sion for them, either doing or not doing routine tests according to their own individual beliefs of what is best.

There is also the question of cost. If a test is necessary it will always be done, but when there is no good evidence that a test will be helpful doctors will think twice about its cost effective-ness. Unfortunately, the National Health Service is not awash with spare money and, like all other specialists, oncologists are under pressure to keep expenses down. So your doctors will want to be sure a test is worthwhile before they recommend it.

Questioning the value of follow up

Perhaps in part because of the cost element, follow up is a part of oncological practice that is currently attracting closer attention. As a result, people are looking critically at what follow up is there for – what does it do? In no particular priority order, the following are some of the arguments that are made in favour of follow up:

- early detection of cancer coming back;
- reassurance;
- picking up late side effects of treatment and helping to deal with them;
- seeing how effective treatment has been;
- research; and
- teaching and training of junior doctors.

These might all seem very reasonable but they are open to debate. Studies have shown that only a very small minority of cancer recurrences are discovered at routine follow up visits. The great majority are diagnosed when people themselves have noticed some new symptom or problem and sought help for this in between their planned outpatient appointments. The evidence suggests that, as far as detecting whether the cancer has come back, it is much more effective to leave this to people to seek attention when they feel they need it, rather than through a scheduled series of clinic visits.

When it comes to reassurance the picture is mixed. Not much research has been done in this area, and almost all of the work that has been published has come from studies of women who have had breast cancer. Some reports have shown that women get a great deal of comfort from their follow up visits, and are pleased to have the regular confirmation that all is well. Others suggest that many women find follow up visits very stressful, with a great deal of anxiety for days or weeks beforehand, being reminded that they have had cancer and worrying about whether 'something bad' will be found when they go for their check up. There are also the practical negatives of a hospital visit: taking time off work, finding someone to look after the children, finding somewhere to park and often waiting ages to be seen for an appointment that may last less than five minutes.

Looking out for longer term side effects of treatment and helping to relieve or control these is important. However, it could once again be argued that this could be done just as well by people asking for appointments as and when they feel they had a problem, rather than by a series of planned visits.

From the doctors' viewpoint, follow-up visits are valuable for seeing what the outcome of treatment has been. If you are offering a particular treatment, then you want to be sure that it is effective and worthwhile. This is even more important in formal research and clinical trials, in which knowing what has happened after treatment is essential in order to make progress and decide whether new therapies are an improvement over existing ones. Likewise, for younger doctors training to be specialists, it is very valuable to see what happens after treatment: checking that the treatment has worked, and learning about any side effects that might occur and how these can be managed. However, all of these benefits are for doctors rather than for the individual person.

A changing pattern?

In the past, follow up after cancer treatment was an almost unthinking ritual, based on practices that were established decades ago. Now its value, how it should be done and who should do it are all being questioned. As yet, however, there are no clearly agreed answers. Follow up is in a state of change. On the one hand, this means that the pattern will vary from hospital to hospital, and from specialist to specialist. However, it also means that doctors are more likely to be flexible about their follow up arrangements, and are more willing to listen to what you want from the process.

Again, in the past, doctors very seldom gave their patients an overview of their follow up care. For instance, explaining why it was being done, how often visits would be arranged, how long they would carry on for and what would happen at those visits was the exception rather than the rule. This is changing, but it is far from universal to be given this information.

A final point worth mentioning is that doctors also vary in what they feel should be included in a follow up consultation. The great majority will tend to focus on your previous cancer, making sure there are no signs of the cancer coming back and no lasting side effects from treatment. Only a minority will broaden the discussion to check on other aspects of your health and wellbeing. In most instances, the likelihood is that if you mention a problem that does not seem to be directly related to your previous cancer, or its treatment, then you will be advised to see your family doctor to look into this, rather than have it dealt with at the oncology clinic.

So, when it comes to follow up it may be helpful for you to take the initiative. Have a think about what you want from the system: would you like the reassurance of regular hospital check ups, or would you find it less stressful to have very occasional visits, say once a year, knowing that if you had problems or worries in between times you could always call for help? Also, who would you like to do your check ups? Would you prefer to go to your hospital specialist (even though you would probably see a member of their team rather than your consultant), or would you rather see a specialist nurse or your GP?

When you have thought through these issues, at your next follow up visit ask about what the plans are for future check ups, and see whether those plans can be adapted to fit with what you would like to happen. See if you can take control of the process, if not actually making the decisions then being involved in the process of how those decisions are agreed.

3

How do I know whether my cancer has come back?

Very understandably, most people's biggest worry after having had treatment for a cancer is 'Will it come back?' As we have seen already, however confident your specialist may be that treatment has been successful, only time will make that certain. However, that may mean a wait of many years to be sure that you are in the clear. For most people anxiety about the cancer coming back lessens as the months and years go by. This decreasing worry is matched by a decrease in risk; the longer things are OK, the more likely it is that you are cured. Most relapses – recurrences of the cancer – happen within the first two or three years after treatment is over, and for most types of cancer the likelihood of a relapse more than five years after treatment is very small indeed.

A rough guide

How do you know if your cancer has come back? What are the signs to look out for? All of us have our off days, when we don't feel so well, with odd twinges and pains, upset tummies or headaches. How do you know when these are just everyday symptoms or when they are signs of the cancer coming back? It can be very difficult to tell, but the following is a useful guideline.

One warning sign may be a symptom, or problem, that you can't easily explain. For example, if you fall off a ladder and hurt your back, and next day you have backache, then there is an obvious cause for your discomfort. However, if you get backache that you haven't had before, without any recent injury or trauma, then that is more of a concern. Also, if that symptom lasts for more than a week without getting any better (most minor health problems will disappear or at least begin to improve after a few days), then you should have a check up with your family doctor. The likelihood is that the check up will find another cause for your problem, rather than confirming a recurrence of your cancer, but it is better to be safe than sorry, and the news that your symptoms were caused by something else will be very reassuring and help to put your mind at rest.

This is very general guidance; is it possible to be a bit more specific about what to look out for? Because there are so many different types of cancer, which can behave in so many different ways, it is impossible to give an overall checklist but I give some more advice that I hope will be helpful.

A bit more detail: local recurrence and distant spread

Cancers usually reappear in one of two ways. They may either develop from traces of the original primary tumour, and so come back as a local recurrence, or they may develop from seedlings of the growth that have spread to other parts of the body, as secondary cancers, or metastases.

If there is a local recurrence, then it is likely to cause similar symptoms to those you had when your cancer was first discovered. For example, if you had a breast cancer, which almost always first appears as a lump in the breast, then finding a new breast lump could be a sign of a local recurrence. Likewise, if you had a prostate cancer, and your original symptoms were difficulty in passing water, a poor stream when you did and having to get up often during the night, then a return of these symptoms might be due to a return of the cancer in your prostate gland.

The reappearance of these symptoms doesn't necessarily mean that your cancer has come back. The breast lump could be a benign cyst or your waterworks problems could be due to non-cancerous changes in your prostate (e.g. there may be narrowing of the urethra, the tube that carries urine through the prostate gland, as a side effect of treatment, or you might be developing a very common condition called benign prostatic hypertrophy, which produces symptoms more or less identical to those with a prostate cancer). The same goes for other types of cancer; a return of your original symptoms, or problems, doesn't always mean that your cancer has come back, but it does mean that you should go and have a check up just to make sure, one way or the other.

When it comes to secondary cancers, the first point to make is that these are not usually scattered out in a haphazard, blunderbuss way, but rather follow a fairly common pattern, depending on the site of the original primary cancer. So, if a prostate cancer spreads, it will almost always go to one or more of the bones in the skeleton; other parts of the body may be affected, but this is much less common. Likewise, if a bowel cancer spreads, it will almost always form metastases in the liver. Sometimes the lungs or other organs in the body may be affected, but the liver is the dominant organ for bowel secondaries. Among the 'big four' cancers, the patterns of secondary spread for breast and lung cancers are less predictable. The bones are most often involved, but spread to the liver, lungs or brain is also very common.

It is also true that although some parts of the body are frequent sites for secondary cancer – the bones, the liver, the lungs and the brain – some other organs are very rarely affected. These include the heart, the pancreas, the stomach, the kidney, the bladder and the small intestine. Why some organs are so often involved and others so rarely remains largely a mystery.

What are the warning signs?

When cancers spread to the bones, the liver, the lungs or the brain, they produce a fairly characteristic set of symptoms. Bone involvement is likely to cause pain at the site of a metastasis, and those metastases are most likely to be in the backbone (the spine) or the pelvis. Liver secondaries may lead to a loss of appetite, a feeling of sickness, pain across the upper part of the belly, loss of weight or jaundice (a yellow colour to the skin and the whites of the eyes). Lung secondaries tend to cause increasing shortness of breath and/or a persistent cough. Brain secondaries may lead to constant headaches, seizures or weakness in certain muscles in the body. All of these symptoms can of course have causes other than cancer. Getting a headache on Sunday afternoon doesn't mean that you've got brain metastases, but getting a headache that is there all the time, hasn't gone away after a week and is getting steadily worse is sinister and needs to be checked out. Likewise, one episode of sickness and vomiting doesn't spell liver secondaries, but feeling more or less constantly nauseated for a week or so is more worrying, and should be investigated.

All this is intended as background information. Every person and every cancer is different. However, if you ask, at the end of your treatment your specialist should be able to tell you the warning signs to look out for in your particular case. The list can't be comprehensive, because no one can predict exactly how any one cancer will behave, but it can give you an idea, if you want it, of the symptoms that you should most be aware to look out for as possible warning signs of a problem.

If your cancer comes back

What happens if your cancer does come back? After months, or even years, of feeling well and getting the 'all clear' at your regular check ups, problems resurface and the tests show that your cancer has returned.

The emotional shock is likely to be enormous. Studies that have tried to measure the impact of the cancer relapse suggest that the news that your cancer is back is even more devastating than when you were first told that you had cancer. The distress is made up of a mixture of many different feelings: disappointment that treatment has failed, anger that it has happened to you, fear about what is going to happen (in terms of what further treatment might be needed and all that that entails) and worry about what the outcome will be – will you get better or have you been handed a death sentence?

Each of us will cope with this news in our own way. It may mean tears, it may mean shouting and cursing, it may mean seeking the comfort and consolation of family and friends, it may mean getting drunk or going back to smoking, or anything else that we think might help, but the amazing point is that nearly everyone does cope. Once the first shock is over, when they have had time to take in the news and absorb what it means, most people will be able to pick up the pieces and move forward. This may not necessarily be with a care-free smile and cheerful optimism but rather with a mixture of resignation and determination to make the best of a bad situation, finding enough positives to make life worth living again and to rebuild your life, taking each day as it comes.

These days, doctors get quite a bit of training about breaking bad news, and usually – but unfortunately not always – you will be told about your relapse in a sensitive and compassionate way, and be given the opportunity both to vent your emotions to the full and then, once you feel ready, to ask all the questions you want to ask. Often, after you have seen your specialist, you will be able to have time with a specialist nurse who can go over matters with you, giving you the chance to talk, to get more information or just to share your feelings and offer you support.

There are no rules for handling this situation; each of us will do it differently. However, once the initial emotional dust has settled, and you have got back a degree of calm, then knowing what your relapse means and what the future holds are among the cornerstones of being able to move forward.

What is the outlook?

The two factors that most influence your outlook are the type of cancer you have and whether it has come back as a local recurrence or as distant metastases – secondary cancers in another part of your body.

If a cancer comes back as a local recurrence, reappearing at the site of your original primary cancer, with some types of cancer further treatment may still be able to produce a cure. For example, if a woman has a breast cancer that is treated with conservative surgery (a lumpectomy followed by radiotherapy, leaving most of her breast intact) and then, a year or two later, the cancer recurs in that breast, it will often be possible to do a mastectomy, removing the remaining breast tissue, which offers a good chance of a cure. In other situations, further surgery, high-dose radiotherapy or chemotherapy might still make a cure possible, or if not they may well be able to control your cancer for a considerable period of time.

If your cancer comes back as distant secondaries, with new tumours in other parts of your body, this unfortunately is usually an incurable situation, but not always. For example, in testicular cancer, even if it has spread widely, chemotherapy still offers a good chance of a complete cure. Also, prospects are improving all the time. For example, as few as ten years or so ago, getting liver secondaries from a bowel cancer (cancer of the colon or rectum) was reckoned to be universally incurable, but now, with improvements in surgery and chemotherapy, some people are being cured.

Despite some positive results, the overall truth is that for most people, if their cancer does come back, then this will be a situation that is ultimately incurable. For many people, however, further treatment with chemotherapy, radiotherapy or, less often, surgery will lead to remission, a period when the cancer will be completely controlled and he or she will be virtually free from any symptoms, feeling more or less completely normal. Furthermore, these remissions often last not just a few weeks or months, but for years. When another relapse does occur, for many cancers further treatment will lead to further remissions, and another lease of life.

So when a cancer comes back a cure may still be possible in some instances. If a cure is not possible, for most people there will be a good chance that further treatment will be able to offer a worthwhile period of relatively normal, comfortable life, and that period of time may well be measured in years. I know that this is a poor second best to the hope of a complete cure, but it is still better than many people imagine when they are first told that their cancer has come back – news that often triggers fears of a very short life expectancy, with a rapid, irreversible and downhill progression.

Usually, but not always, your specialists will have a good idea of what the likely long-term outcome will be if your cancer does come back. They won't be able to give you a precise timetable, but they will be able to tell you if there is a chance of a cure, and how good that chance is, and if there is not then what an average life expectancy might be, and what will be needed in the way of treatment. Curability and life expectancy are very sensitive and emotive subjects, and your specialist is likely to wait for you to ask the questions rather than force the information on you, but usually if you do ask they will give you an honest and frank reply, based on their knowledge and experience. Remember, however, that they do not have a crystal ball. They can only tell you what is likely to happen, and each of us is different – there will always be exceptions to every rule.

4
Side effects of treatment

There are countless possible side effects of cancer treatment, and it is impossible to describe them all in a book of this length. Later in this chapter we look at a few specific problems in a little more detail, but my main aim is to cover some general principles about side effects and what can and cannot be done about them.

Back in the 1970s a new chemotherapy treatment was introduced for testicular cancer. It was called BEP and was a cocktail of three drugs: bleomycin, etoposide and (cis)platinum. Overnight, it transformed the outlook for advanced testicular cancer – a condition that had previously been universally incurable became almost universally curable. This dramatic improvement in outcome came at a price, however: BEP caused horrendous sickness, and this was before the days of modern day anti-sickness drugs. I remember being at a meeting in New York when one of the pioneers of BEP was describing his results. When it came to questions afterward, someone asked 'How do you control the nausea and vomiting?' 'We can't,' was the reply, and the speaker added 'so I tell the guy, you can have the chemo, be sick as a dog for four months and be cured, or you can go out on the sidewalk and die. I find they choose the chemo.' The point of this story is that the achievements in improving cure rates with cancer treatment have been truly dramatic over the past 50 years, but many of those cures have come at a price, and that price is toxicity: side effects. In the main, medical attention has been focused on the chances of cure, or increased survival, with less of an emphasis on the side effects.

Surely if certain death in a matter of months can be turned into another ten years or more of life by a course of treatment, then a few side effects are a small price to pay – after all, you never get something for nothing.

When rapid progress is being made, when remissions that were never possible previously suddenly become routine, this concentration on the benefits of treatment and relative neglect of its downsides is understandable, especially if those downsides are short term. Yes, if you have chemotherapy you may lose your hair and you may be sick, but once the treatment is over your hair grows back, the sickness stops and you are alive! However, with the passage of time this philosophy is changing, with an increasing emphasis on trying to reduce or control side effects, and a realization that with some treatments side effects are not just a short-term nuisance but can go on to become a long-term if not permanent problem.

Side effects differ in when they occur. In the past, most attention was given to the immediate, short-term toxicities of treatment. These can be dramatic and distressing: tiredness, sickness, hair loss, pain, infection and so on – the list is considerable. However, these problems are 'immediate' and 'short term'. Even if they cannot be fully controlled, they will usually disappear fairly rapidly once the treatment is over, but there are other possible side effects that may appear months, or even years, after treatment is complete. These tend to be much more difficult to manage, and are often long-term or even permanent complications.

What causes long-term side effects?

The biological processes that lead to these long-term complications of treatment are many and complex, but the following is a very crude explanation of the pathological process that underlies many of them. The major cancer therapies – surgery, radiotherapy and chemotherapy – all have the potential to cause inflammation in the organs or tissues where a tumour is present. This inflammation may simply settle and disappear over time, but on other occasions it will cause permanent damage to small blood vessels in the area and this will lead to some of the normal tissue that has been affected being replaced by scar tissue. This process is sometimes called fibrosis. Fibrosis doesn't happen overnight. It is a slow process that evolves over many months or years; it may be five to ten years after treatment before it is complete. Once it has occurred it is permanent; there is no magic bullet that will get rid of it. Occasionally, surgery may be able to remove it, but this is the rare exception and not the rule.

Whether sufficient fibrosis will occur to cause long-term side effects depends on a number of factors. The type and extent of treatment form one variable; having high-dose radiotherapy or very major surgery are both likely to lead to considerable scar tissue formation in the area of the body that has been treated. Also, some organs are more vulnerable than others. For example, organs such as the kidneys, the lungs, the small intestine and the liver are very sensitive to radiation, and can be permanently damaged by relatively low doses, whereas other organs such as the brain, the bladder and the skin can tolerate much higher doses before they are irreversibly injured.

Then there is the mystery of individual variation. Suppose two people who are apparently very similar in age and general fitness, with identical types of cancer, undergo exactly the same treatment; one may have no long-term problems, whereas the other may go on to develop significant permanent complications. Why this should be remains, in most instances, a puzzle, and in most instances there is no way to predict in advance who will or will not develop long-term difficulties.

For example, after curative radiotherapy for early cancer of the prostate, about one in 20 men will develop some degree of permanent damage to their rectum. This is because the rectum, the lowermost part of the large bowel, lies up against the prostate gland and inevitably receives quite a high dose of radiation. However, there is no way that doctors can test for this individual sensitivity and work out in advance who will or will not go on to develop long-term rectal problems, which can lead to chronic diarrhoea, pain and bleeding from the back passage. In the same way, about one in 20 women who have surgery for breast cancer that involves complete removal of the lymph nodes in their armpit (what surgeons call a total axillary clearance) will go on to develop some degree of lymphoedema – swelling of the arm on the same side that the surgery has been performed. Why a few women develop this complication when the great majority, having apparently identical surgery, do not remains unclear. Unfortunately, then, whether you have long-term side effects as a result of your cancer treatment is to some extent a lottery.

Timing and duration of side effects

Doctors talk about side effects as being either short term, medium term or long term. Exactly what these mean in terms of time isn't precisely defined, but short-term side effects can usually be expected to last anywhere from a few days to a few weeks, medium-term problems can be measured in months and the long-term ones in years.

Nearly everyone will have some short-term side effects from his or her cancer treatment. After surgery, there will be some temporary pain or discomfort; after radiotherapy there will be some local inflammation of the part of the body that was irradiated; and after chemotherapy, sickness, the risk of infection and hair loss are common problems. With all of these therapies, there will be some temporary tiredness and loss of energy. For most people, however, most of these upsets settle within a few weeks of the treatment being over, if not before. Also, at this time, although treatment is continuing or in its immediate aftermath, hospital visits, medical and nursing support will be fairly intensive, and any side effects that do develop will usually get prompt and effective attention. Pain killers will be given for discomfort, anti-emetic drugs prescribed for sickness, antibiotics for infection and so on. Every effort will be made by your clinical team to keep you as comfortable as possible.

Once treatment is over, those hospital visits become less frequent and the support of the clinical team is often less readily available. Generally, this isn't too great a difficulty. Those people who do have ongoing side effects will still be seen regularly until they have fully resolved. Also, it is always possible to phone for an earlier appointment if you are worried.

However, something that can be confusing and puzzling is the appearance of long-term side effects. This is because these can often develop many months, or even years, after treatment is over. Life gets more or less back to normal, you've been feeling quite well and then you become aware of a new health problem. Depending on your symptoms, it may or may not occur to you that this could be related to your previous cancer and its treatment.

Deciding what to do about this is not always easy. As I stated previously, all of us have our 'off days' when we have odd aches and pains, or just feel generally unwell, and going to see your family doctor or specialist every time this happens runs the risk of getting you labelled as over-anxious, so that if anything serious does crop up it might be missed. On the other hand, you don't want to run the risk of ignoring a problem that, if not diagnosed and treated, could cause you ongoing distress and might even be dangerous. My advice here goes back to what I said earlier. If you get a new symptom or problem that you cannot readily explain, and it lasts more than about a week, without any sign of getting better, then you should seek your doctor's advice about it.

When you do see either your family doctor or your specialist, there are at least four possible outcomes. One is that they will be able to reassure you that there is nothing to worry about. The second is that they may diagnose some medical condition completely unrelated to your previous cancer and its treatment. The third is that they may find evidence to suggest that your cancer has come back or spread. Finally, they may decide that you have developed a long-term side effect of your original treatment.

Incidentally, sometimes it can be very difficult to tell whether a new health problem is due to your cancer coming back or to long-term side effects; the pattern of symptoms can often be very similar. Also, you may need a number of tests and investigations before your doctors can be totally sure about what is wrong.

With this background knowledge, we can now go on to look at a couple of the more common long-term side effects of treatment that can occur.

Tiredness: cancer-related fatigue

This is the most common after effect of cancer treatment; it has been estimated that more than eight out of ten people having chemotherapy, or curative, high-dose radiotherapy will experience it to some degree.

We all have days when we feel tired, but the tiredness linked to cancer and its treatment is much more than this. It is a constant feeling of tiredness, weakness and lack of energy that interferes with day to day living. Importantly, and in contrast to everyday tiredness, it isn't helped by resting or sleeping: you feel just as exhausted after a good night's sleep as you did before. Perhaps because tiredness is so common, it has taken doctors a long time to appreciate how important a problem it is for people with cancer. Until a few years ago textbooks hardly mentioned it, and research into its causes and treatment is still at a relatively early stage, but now it has been clearly recognized by oncologists as a major side effect of cancer and its treatment, and acknowledged as something that is much more troublesome than 'ordinary' tiredness. To make this distinction clear, they have coined the phrase 'cancer-related fatigue' (CRF) to describe it.

CRF can be caused both by the cancer itself and as a side effect of treatment. Research suggests that about four out of ten people diagnosed with cancer will have CRF before they actually start their treatment. However, eight or more out of ten people having chemotherapy or a course of radiotherapy will experience the problem, and it is also common with other types of treatment, such as hormone therapy and some surgical operations. For many people, CRF will settle quite quickly once treatment is finished, but for about one in three it will last for months or even years. Most of the limited amount of research into the problem conducted to date has looked at women with breast cancer, and this has shown that 35 per cent, more than three out of ten, women developed CRF that lasted for more than a year after their cancer was diagnosed, and as many as one in five experienced it for more than five years. There is some evidence that the older you are, the more likely you are to get CRF, and that it will last longer than in younger people. Also, if you have CRF before you start treatment, then it is more likely to continue after your treatment is over.

Exactly what causes CRF remains a mystery, but a great deal of research is being done to try and discover more about it. One important point is that having CRF after your cancer treatment doesn't mean you still have cancer. Many people who are completely cured will have CRF for months or years after their treatment is over.

Can anything be done to help? The answer, very often, is that yes it can, but the first step is to get your medical team to realize that you have a problem, that you have CRF and not just 'a bit of tiredness'. CRF is now recognized as being often more distressing and disruptive than any other side effect of cancer treatment, with more than nine out of ten people who have it saying that it interferes with day to day living, such that they have to change their everyday routine to cope with it. Even basic tasks like preparing simple meals, doing a bit of light housework or socializing with friends and family can become a real burden. It also causes problems for people who are working. Often, they need time off work or have to reduce their hours or change what they do; sometimes their partners may need to take time off to help them cope, or they may have to employ someone to do chores at home that they cannot manage, all of which can cause financial problems. These days there are a number of questionnaires, and rating scales, that can help doctors decide when someone has CRF, so if tiredness after your cancer is a problem for you then do discuss it with your specialist. If they don't know about it they can't be expected to help, so the first step toward improvement is letting them know that you do have a problem.

Unfortunately, although researchers are looking for one, there isn't a single magic pill or treatment that will get rid of CRF. Until someone discovers a single treatable cause for the problem, the approach to managing the condition will continue to be based on the belief that there are probably a number of different causes that can contribute to the syndrome and looking for these, and that treating them if they are present is the best way forward. Brief discussions of some of the possible causes of CRF, as well as potential ways to manage them, are given below.

Anaemia

Being anaemic – having a low level of haemoglobin in your blood – is a very common problem after cancer treatment. It may be the result either of having had the cancer or it may be a side effect of treatment. Being anaemic makes you feel tired.

It can also make you breathless and lead to a feeling of general weakness. A simple blood test will tell whether you are anaemic. If you are, then this is usually easy to correct. Depending on the type of anaemia you have, this may mean something as simple as taking some iron tablets for a few weeks, or it may mean something more complicated like a blood transfusion (usually done over a few hours as an outpatient, and giving an almost instant dramatic improvement in how you feel) or a course of injections to stimulate your bone marrow to make more blood cells.

Pain

If you have pain that is uncontrolled, or poorly controlled, this can be very wearing and energy sapping. Your doctors will only know if you have pain if you tell them, so if it is a problem do let them know. With modern day pain killers, nearly all cancer related pain, and cancer treatment related pain, can be easily and safely controlled.

Depression and anxiety

Cancer and its treatment are closely linked to anxiety and depression; worries about the cancer and whether it will come back, the disruption to your life caused by the diagnosis and treatment of your cancer can amount to an enormous emotional burden. For many people this will tip them over into clinical anxiety states or depression, which can be helped by simple and safe drug treatment. Many people worry about taking drugs if they are anxious or depressed, but very often a short course of treatment can break the cycle of these mood altering states, which can come to dominate life and can be very hard to escape from without medical help.

Sleep disorders

Sleeping poorly is a common difficulty after cancer treatment, and not getting enough sleep will make any existing tiredness worse. If this is a problem for you, talk it through with your doctors or nurses. It may be that some sleeping tablets would help, but often they will be able to give other advice to help ease your insomnia, like having a relaxing bath and a hot milky drink before you go to bed.

Other medical problems

Sometimes cancer, or its treatment, can bring to light other medical problems that weren't obvious beforehand, such as diabetes or low thyroid function (myxoedema), or there may be direct medical complications of treatment affecting heart or lung function that may make tiredness more likely. Part of the medical checks for someone with CRF will often include some simple tests to make sure that none of these other problems are present and contributing to your tiredness. If those tests do bring any of these problems to light, then obviously they can be treated appropriately, which should help to make you feel better.

Diet

Not eating the right foods, not feeling like eating or not being able to eat properly for some reason can add to feelings of tiredness. If you are experiencing any eating problems or have any concerns about your diet, do mention them to you medical team; they will either offer advice themselves or arrange for you to see an expert dietician who might be able to help you.

Exercise

If you are feeling exhausted, talking about exercise may seem rather ridiculous. However, there is good evidence that for many people with CRF some gentle exercise can help to improve their symptoms and give them back some energy. This doesn't mean running the half marathon, or doing 20 press ups, but just a slight increase in activity can often make a difference. Once again, mention this to your medical team and if you need help they may be able to arrange expert advice from a physiotherapist or occupational therapist to advise you about what is best for you.

Complementary therapies

These days countless complementary therapies are available; mostly these have to be arranged privately, but occasionally they are available on the National Health Service. Many doctors remain sceptical about the benefits of these therapies, feeling that they have not been properly tested in clinical trials, but many people find them very comforting and life enhancing. Meditation, reflexology, aromatherapy and massage, music therapy and relaxation are among a number of different therapies that people with CRF may find helpful. What people find beneficial is very much a matter of personal choice, and it is difficult to make any firm recommendations.

Lymphoedema

Lymphoedema is a gradual build up of fluid (lymph) in part of the body caused by surgical removal of or radiotherapy damage to nearby lymph nodes. It is most often seen in women who have had breast cancer, who have needed surgery or radiotherapy to the lymph nodes in their armpit (the axillary lymph nodes). Following this treatment, about one in 20 women will go on to get some swelling of the arm on the side that has been affected. However, lymphoedema can also develop in the legs if surgery or radiotherapy has been necessary to treat lymph nodes in the groin or pelvis, and rarely it can affect other parts of the body. It comes on gradually after the end of treatment, appearing anywhere from one to five years later. Very often the changes are slight, with the arm or leg feeling a bit fuller or heavier, and some mild tightness or stretching of the skin. Sometimes, however, the build up of fluid can be considerable, leading to very obvious swelling of the limb, which in turn causes pain and stiffness, together with thickening of the skin and underlying tissues (doctors often call this brawny oedema).

The risk of getting lymphoedema, and the severity of the problem, relate mainly to the extent of treatment to the lymph nodes. These nodes form part of the lymphatic system and help to drain fluid from the arm or leg, through the network of lymph vessels that run throughout the tissues. Both surgery and radiotherapy can damage this drainage system, reducing the flow of lymph and so causing a build up of fluid in the limb. Lymphoedema is more likely to appear if both surgery and radiotherapy are used to treat a particular group of lymph nodes, but occasionally it can develop after only relatively minor treatment. It is not always possible to predict who will or will not get lymphoedema. Unfortunately, the changes in the tissues that cause lymphoedema cannot be reversed, so once the condition develops it is permanent.

Although it cannot be reversed, much can be done to control lymphoedema if it develops. Nowadays, most hospitals will have links to lymphoedema clinics, where specialist teams can advise on care of the condition. Depending on the severity of the problem, this might involve a number of different measures, including the following:

- information on how to look after the skin of the affected limb, with use of a regular moisturizer, protecting the skin against minor injury and avoiding sunburn;
- fitting an elasticated sleeve that can be worn, possibly all the time, on the affected limb, which helps to control the swelling and eases discomfort;

- teaching manual lymphatic drainage – a form of massage that helps to move lymph fluid out of the swollen limb;
- bandaging – a more intensive therapy that involves regular, quite tight bandages being applied to the limb; usually, an expert is required to carry out the treatment; and
- the use of vacuum pumps – sleeves that fit over the limb and are connected to a motor that creates pressure in the sleeve, helping to push fluid out of the limb.

A number of the national cancer charities in the UK, including Cancerbackup and Breast Cancer Care, have detailed booklets and information on lymphoedema and its management.

5

What can I do to stop my cancer coming back?

However vigorous the reassurances from your medical team that your chances of a cure are very good, there will be times when nagging doubts creep in. Being aware of the possible warning signs that could signal a return of your cancer is a help. If you haven't got any of the symptoms then everything is probably OK, and if you do develop a problem you know you should quickly get it checked out, but can you be more proactive? Is there anything you can do positively to reduce the risk of your cancer coming back? Up to a point the answer is yes, and in this chapter we will explore some of the possible options.

Lifestyle and cancer risk

Experts suggest that anywhere from a one-quarter to three-quarters of all cancers are the result of aspects of our own lifestyle, which we can control and are responsible for. These include whether we smoke, our weight, what we eat and drink, our levels of physical activity and, if you are a woman, whether you use hormone replacement therapy (HRT). If one or more of these was a factor in the development of your cancer, a change in lifestyle could well help to reduce your risk of a relapse. Even if your medical team don't think any of these contributed to your original cancer, but you know that one or more of them form part of your everyday pattern of life, making a change could still reduce your chances of getting another type of cancer in the future.

Smoking

Nearly everyone knows that smoking is the major cause of lung cancer, but smoking increases the risk of getting a range of other cancers, including bladder cancer, cancers of the mouth and throat, cancer of the pancreas and cancer of the cervix. Of course, there are also the other smoking-related diseases to consider, including chronic bronchitis, emphysema and heart disease, all of which can be fatal. The bottom line of these medical hazards is that one out of every two people who smoke more than 20 cigarettes a day will die from a smoking related-disease.

An important point to remember is that if you have had a smoking-related cancer, and have had that treated, this unfortunately doesn't protect you from getting further cancers in the future. For example, if someone gets an early cancer of the vocal cords as a result of smoking, treatment is likely to be successful because this is a highly curable cancer. However, if the person continues to smoke, he or she will still be at a much greater risk than nonsmokers of getting lung cancer, bladder cancer or cancer of the pancreas.

If you are a smoker and you stop, this will reduce your risk of getting cancer. Overall, your chances of getting a lung cancer will have halved after ten years of not smoking. The longer you stop smoking, the lower your risk. Even if you are in your fifties, and have been a lifelong smoker, stopping can more than halve your chance of getting a lung cancer. Another set of statistics that might encourage smokers to give up is that on average people who stop when they are 30 years old have an extra ten years of life compared with those who carry on smoking, and even if they only stop when they're 60 years old they still gain three extra years. It is never too late to stop.

What about 'half-measures'? Suppose you cut back or change to a pipe or cigars? There is some evidence that reducing the number of cigarettes you smoke each day helps a bit, but only a bit. The figures are that if you followed 100 lifelong smokers of 20 a day, then by the age of 75 years 50 of them would have developed lung cancer; by reducing to 10 cigarettes or less each day, the number of cancers would reduce to about 37. You've slightly reduced the odds but there's still a better than one in three chance that you'll end up with lung cancer. Changing to a pipe or cigars is a slightly more effective way of reducing your risk; you will be about 50 per cent less likely to develop lung cancer than a heavy smoker, but that risk is still almost 50 per cent more than that for a nonsmoker. Cutting back or changing to cigars or a pipe are half-measures, or even less than 'half' measures. If you can, it is far better to give up completely, but that is easier said than done.

Surveys suggest that almost three out of four smokers would like to quit, and more than half say they intend to do so in the next 12 months. The stronger the desire, the greater the chance of success, but if you do want to stop you are probably going to need help. Research suggests that using will power alone, only about one in 30 smokers who want to stop actually will. The two main approaches to backing up personal motivation, supporting your desire to stop, are counselling and medication.

Counselling, or intensive behavioural support, has been shown to work; about one in ten smokers who go through the course will manage to give up the habit. The courses are run by specially trained smoking cessation counsellors. In the UK, counselling services to help people give up smoking are now available on the National Health Service (NHS), and your family doctor should be able to arrange this for you.

Medication to help people give up smoking comes in two main types: nicotine replacement therapy and drugs called Zyban (buproprion) and Champix (verenicline). Like counselling, about one in ten smokers who want to give up, and use nicotine replacement therapy to help them, find that they succeed.

Nicotine replacement therapy comes in a number of forms: you can chew it as a gum; stick it on your skin as a transdermal patch; suck it as a lozenge; squirt it up your nose as a nasal spray; take it as a tablet that you put under your tongue and allow to dissolve; or inhale it from a puffer (like those used by people with asthma). All forms of nicotine replacement therapy are now available on prescription on the NHS, or – if you prefer – the patches, gum and lozenges can all be bought over the counter at pharmacists or supermarkets.

Zyban is a drug that was originally developed as an anti-depressant. When it was being tested in clinical trials it was realized that it also reduced people's need to smoke. Zyban is available on prescription on the NHS in the UK. Another tablet, Champix, has also been approved in the UK. Studies show this to be effective, or even more effective, than Zyban at reducing the craving for cigarettes. Champix is taken once or twice a day and, like Zyban, is available on prescription.

Counselling and medication can be used together, and studies suggest that combining them does help, with as many as one in five smokers being able to give up as a result.

If you are thinking of giving up (and please do), the NHS is keen to help and strongly supports smokers who want to stop; it spent more than £50 million on its Stop Smoking Services in 2006. A first step would be either to see your family doctor, who can give you advice about planning your campaign, put you in touch with counselling services and arrange prescriptions for medications if you need them. Or you could phone the NHS smoking helpline (0800 1690 169). Do give it a try; you would be doing yourself a favour, with a real chance of improving your health and reducing the risk of a previous smoking-related cancer coming back and the chances of developing a new one. There is also the bonus that you would save yourself a great deal of money.

Being overweight and cancer risk

The evidence that being overweight increases our risk of getting cancer is overwhelming. Estimates suggest that as many as one in five cancers in women, and slightly fewer in men, could be caused by being too heavy. Put another way, in the UK every year more than 10,000 new cancers are due to people not having a healthy body weight, but this isn't generally known. A survey by the American Cancer Society recently showed that fewer than one in 20 people knew that being overweight increased their chance of getting cancer. Likewise, a European study asking men about the hazards of being too heavy showed that although four out of ten knew about heart disease or diabetes, cancer was not mentioned.

The link between being overweight and developing cancer was first recognized in cancer of the womb (endometrial cancer). Each year more than 4,500 women in the UK will be told that they have cancer of the womb, which makes it the fifth commonest cancer in women. Although most of those women will be cured, there are still about 900 deaths each year from the disease. The evidence is that as many as four out of every ten cases of cancer of the womb are caused by being overweight; studies have shown that a woman in her late fifties who is overweight, or obese, is five times more likely than other women to get endometrial cancer. Also, the more weight gained, the greater the risk; for example, if you are 50 pounds (22.7 kilograms) or more overweight then you are ten times more likely to get womb cancer than women of normal weight.

Breast cancer is another cancer in which women who are past the menopause, and overweight, are at greater risk than those of the same age whose weight is in the normal range. Estimates suggest that almost one in ten breast cancers is caused by being overweight. The good news is that studies have shown that women who are able to lose weight after the menopause actually reduce their chances of getting breast cancer.

Men are also at risk from being too heavy. Studies suggest that about one in 20 prostate cancers are caused by being overweight. Of those cancers that affect both men and women, about one in ten colon cancers and as many as one in four cancers of the kidney are linked to being overweight or obese. There is also evidence that people who are obese and develop colon cancer, kidney cancer, or cancer of the gullet (oesophagus) or pancreas are more likely to die from their cancer than people of normal weight.

All of these statistics come mainly from research looking at what has caused cancer in the first place, rather than what causes a cancer to come back after treatment. There is, however, a growing body of evidence to suggest that being overweight, or obese, does increase your risk of a relapse after you have had apparently curative therapy. Studies in people who have had breast cancer, bowel cancer or prostate cancer have all shown that those who are considerably overweight, or obese, are at greater risk of their cancer coming back than people who are of normal weight. The figures vary in different studies but people who are obese seem to be between one-third to a half more likely to have their cancer come back, than someone who is of normal weight. To put these numbers another way, if ten out of every 100 people of normal weight relapsed, then for people who are obese 13 to 15 would have their cancer come back.

Just jumping on the scales or looking in the mirror does not necessarily tell you if you are overweight or how overweight you are, although it might give you a strong clue. The accurate measure is called the body mass index (BMI). You can work out your BMI by measuring your weight (in kilograms) and your height (in metres); you then divide your weight by the square of your height. According to World Health Organization guide-lines, if the answer comes out below 25 then your weight is normal; if it is between 25 and 30 you are overweight; and if it is over 30 you are obese. Unfortunately, the formula is a bit complicated, and most of us in the UK still think in imperial rather than metric measurements, so an example might help. If a man, or woman, is five feet and seven inches tall, and weighs 10.5 stones, then their BMI is normal; if they weigh 12.5 stones then they will be overweight; and if they weigh 14.5 stones then they will be obese.

If you think that you are overweight, ask your medical team to check out your BMI. If their figures confirm that there is a problem, then ask their advice about losing weight. If they think it is a good idea, and might help you to reduce your risk of your cancer coming back or getting other health problems, then they should be able to arrange for you to see an expert dietician who can give you advice on how best to shed the pounds.

Diet: what we eat and the risk of cancer

There is probably more written about what we eat and how it relates to cancer than about any other possible causes of the disease. Unfortunately, a vast number of these reports are unreliable, irrelevant or both. They are hugely popular with the media, however, and any publication in a scientific journal that links a food or drink to cancer is bound to get its quota of column inches in one or more national newspapers.

Once again, most of the information on this subject comes from research into what causes cancer in the first place, rather than what helps to stop it coming back after treatment. From these studies, the strongest link is between eating red meat and getting bowel cancer (and, to a lesser extent, prostate cancer). The pooled results from a number of reports suggest that eating on average more than 100 to 120 grams of red meat each day increases your risk of bowel cancer by about 25 per cent, and eating more than 30 grams of processed red meat (such as sausages, pates and pies) each day increases your risk by 30 to 50 per cent. Based on these figures, although the overall chance of getting bowel cancer is two per cent (i.e. it will affect one person in 50), among people who eat large amounts of red meat regularly that figure falls to about one in 25 to 35; the odds have shortened and the risk is increased. Other studies have also suggested that a diet rich in red meat or processed red meat could also increase the risk of breast cancer and stomach cancer, but there are fewer reports about these cancers and the evidence base is not as strong as that for bowel cancer, although this could change with time. However, these results do support the general message that too much red meat or red meat products may increase your cancer risk.

Another quite strong link, this time a positive one, is between lycopenes and reducing your risk of prostate cancer. Lycopene is a protein found in tomatoes, and it becomes even more concentrated when tomatoes are processed or cooked with oil. Lycopene is a potent antioxidant, and the general opinion is that antioxidants are good when it comes to trying to reduce our cancer risk.

It is important to mention that the likelihood of our foods increasing or reducing our risk of getting cancer depends not only on what we eat and how much, but also on how often we have them. Eating one steak won't give you bowel cancer, and eating two tomatoes won't prevent you from getting prostate cancer. We are talking about regular consumption of specific foods over a long period of time. This is another point that often isn't made clear in media coverage of scientific reports on the subject.

Incidentally, researchers have found that when it comes to diet and health, people are far happier to take some sort of supplement to add to what they eat normally than actually to change what they are eating. Understandably, this has led to a great deal of research about the role of vitamin supplements in cancer prevention. The literature is vast, and the results of individual studies often give contradictory answers; some claim to show great benefits, others show no effect and others still show positive harm, with an actual increase in the number of cancers. The overall result is that there is no good evidence that taking regular vitamin supplements helps to reduce our risk of getting cancer or lessens the chances of it coming back after treatment.

The limited research that has been done on the link between diet and cancer relapse has mainly involved women who have had breast cancer, but the findings support the other results, showing that a diet rich in fruit and vegetables and low in salt and fat reduces the risk of the cancer coming back.

On balance, looking at the detail of what we eat in our diets and trying to pick individual foods that will reduce our risk of cancer isn't terribly helpful. The best overall advice is to have plenty of fresh fruit and vegetables, and to keep portions of red meat, especially processed meat, to two or three per week. This not only will match with what evidence there is for the risks and benefits of diet and cancer formation, but will fit in with the far stronger evidence for the link between a healthy diet and reduction in heart disease and diabetes.

Alcohol

The link between drinking alcohol and getting cancer is complicated. It is also regularly highlighted by the media, often in very alarmist ways, when any new scientific report on the subject appears. The evidence is that there are some cancers that are more likely to occur in moderate or heavy drinkers, and there are other cancers for which there is no evidence of such an increased risk.

The clearest evidence of a link between drinking alcohol and cancer comes from people with cancers of the throat (pharynx) and voice box (larynx), but these are quite uncommon and together make up only about one per cent of all cancers. Among the common cancers, the two for which there is most evidence of a link to alcohol are large bowel cancer and breast cancer.

In cancer of the large bowel (the colon or the rectum), moderate or heavy drinkers are about ten per cent more likely than nondrinkers to develop one of these tumours. This may sound alarming, but putting the statistics another way it means that among every 1,000 'normal' people, about 20 will develop a bowel cancer at some time during their life, but among heavy drinkers that number would rise to 22 in every 1,000. This is still an increase, but it certainly does not suggest that every heavy drinker will get bowel cancer. The link between alcohol and breast cancer is one that has attracted much publicity in recent years. The research suggests that, overall, in every 1,000 women about 110 will develop breast cancer. Among women who are moderate drinkers that figure would rise to about 117, and among heavy drinkers it may be as high as 130 to 140 out of every 1,000. Although this is still an increase, it is less frightening than the media often suggest.

Other cancers for which there is some evidence that regular drinking makes them more likely include liver cancer and cancer of the gullet (cancer of the oesophagus). On the other hand, research has failed to identify any link between alcohol and a number of other more common cancers, such as prostate cancer and cancer of the ovary.

These figures all relate to preventing cancer developing in the first place, and virtually no research has been done to evaluate the effects of drinking alcohol on cancer recurrence. There is also the other side of the argument, which suggests that a modest amount of alcohol might actually help to protect against heart disease. So, although there is no doubt that heavy drinking is harmful, there is good evidence that people who drink the equivalent of a glass of wine each day have a better life expectancy than nondrinkers. When it comes to reducing your risk of cancer recurrence, there really isn't sufficient evidence to make a recommendation either way, but heavy drinking and binge drinking are bad for your general health and the safest thing to do is keep within the UK Government advice. This advice indicates that a woman should drink no more than 14 units each week, and a man no more than 21 units (one unit being equal to eight grams of alcohol; this is roughly the same as a small [125ml] glass of wine, or a pint of beer, or a single measure of spirits).

The importance of exercise

How much we weigh is clearly due to how much we eat, but it also depends on how much we exercise – how much physical activity we do to burn off the calories. Although few people realize it, regular exercise can help to reduce our risk of getting cancer and, very importantly, it has also clearly been shown to reduce the chances of cancer coming back after treatment.

Different studies looking at people who have had bowel cancer, prostate cancer, lung cancer or breast cancer all show that taking regular exercise reduced their chances of their cancer coming back by more than one-third. For example in the study on bowel cancer, three years after finishing treatment 25% (one in four) of those who took little or no exercise had relapsed, but in the group of people who exercised regularly the cancer had returned in only 15% (fewer than one in six), so the chance of the cancer coming back was reduced by more than a third. The most dramatic findings come from a recent study of breast cancer survivors, looking at the effects of diet and exercise, in which the researchers found that eating at least five servings of vegetables and fruit a day and doing exercise equivalent to walking briskly for 30 minutes, six days a week, reduced the risk of dying from recurrent breast cancer by 50 per cent. In other words, a sensible diet and regular moderate exercise could halve your likelihood of your cancer coming back.

Exactly why regular exercise can help prevent cancer remains uncertain. It could just be that people who are more physically active lead a generally more healthy lifestyle, but there are also scientific findings showing that the levels of a number of growth factors, circulating in the blood, which could cause cells to become cancerous are reduced in people who are more active.

One encouraging point from the research is that there is no proof that very vigorous exercise has any extra benefit over just those few hours of brisk walking each week. So you don't have to push yourself to the limit.

Exercise helps us to keep fit in other ways, and it certainly reduces the risk of heart disease, which is an even bigger killer than cancer. It also improves the quality of life, reducing tiredness and boosting wellbeing and self-esteem. For some time now the UK Government has recommended the brisk walking regimen – 30 to 40 minutes on five days per week, or its equivalent – as a key part of a healthy lifestyle. However, official figures suggest only a quarter of women, and just over a third of men, manage even this modest target. It doesn't take a lot to make a difference – walking up stairs rather than taking lifts or escalators, walking to the shops instead of getting into the car, or going for a turn round the park or along the canal towpath. A mile or two a day helps keep the cancer away!

Hormone replacement therapy

A huge amount of research has been done to try to work out whether taking HRT is a cancer risk, and the answers aren't simple. There is good evidence that taking HRT when you are over 50 increases your risk of developing breast cancer, ovarian cancer and cancer of the womb, but there is also evidence that it reduces a woman's risk of getting bowel cancer.

For women who have had cancer and are concerned about taking HRT, the clearest findings are in breast cancer where there is now strong evidence that taking HRT does increase your chances of the cancer coming back. To put this into context, the figures from the latest trial to be published (in April 2008) suggest that five years after treatment, among women who continue to take HRT there will be twice as many relapses as in those who don't (about 20 per cent compared with only about 10 per cent). These results, when added to the findings from previous studies, strongly support the recommendation that a woman who has had breast cancer should not take HRT.

For women who have had other types of cancer and are worried about their cancer coming back, there is very little evidence on which to base firm advice. Also, most women don't take HRT for fun. Usually, it is given to help them to cope with menopausal symptoms, such as hot flushes, night sweats, loss of libido, vaginal dryness and so on. For some women these are very minor problems, but for others they can be hugely distressing, even driving them to the brink of suicide. So, at the end of the day, whether to have HRT is a matter of weighing up the risks and the benefits. If the hot flushes are ruining your life, making you clinically depressed and raising thoughts of ending it all, then a slight increase in the possibility of your cancer coming back may be a minor consideration, and HRT might be the answer. However, if your symptoms aren't really much bother then avoid it. If you are concerned, and in doubt, the thing to do is to have a chat with your family doctor; they can help you to weigh up your individual pros and cons, so that you can reach an agreed and informed decision on what to do.

If you are having problems with menopausal symptoms, then one organization that it might be helpful to know about is The Daisy Network: Premature Menopause Support Group. This offers a confidential service for women who have had an early menopause, allowing them to share their experience; it also gives a list of helpful books. Postal address details are as follows: PO BOX 183, Rossendale, Lancashire, BB4 6WZ. The website is <www.daisynetwork.org.uk>.

Lifestyle and quality of life

Although advice on how to lead a healthy lifestyle is widely available, and regularly publicized in the media, not everyone takes up the message. In May 2008 the *Journal of Clinical Oncology* published a survey looking at more than 9,000 survivors of different types of cancer (breast cancer, prostate cancer, bowel cancer, bladder cancer, cancer of the womb and malignant melanoma). The researchers had asked people if they ate an average of five or more portions of fruit and vegetables a day, whether they took regular exercise and whether they smoked. The good news was that about nine out of ten were nonsmokers or had given up smoking. When it came to diet and exercise the figures were less encouraging; only about one in three took regular physical exercise, and fewer than one in five managed the 5-A-Day fruit and vegetable diet. Only one in 20 managed all three lifestyle recommendations. However, the researchers also discovered that the closer people came to meeting those three health goals, the better was their overall quality of life. This was a North American study, but almost certainly the results would be similar in the UK and they do strongly suggest that leading a healthy lifestyle is not only 'good for you' but actually makes you feel better too.

Keep taking the tablets

For the past 30 years or so, women with hormone sensitive (oestrogen receptor positive) breast cancer have very often been given the tablet tamoxifen to take for five years or more after their initial treatment was over, in order to reduce their risk of their cancer coming back. More recently a new group of drugs, called aromatase inhibitors, have also been used in this way to reduce the risk of relapse in breast cancer (these include the drugs anastrozole [Armidex], letrozole [Femara] and exemestane [Aromasin]). For some people who have had bowel cancer, the drug capecitabine (Xeloda) is also being given as a tablet for a year or so after treatment, to help to reduce the risk of a recurrence. The likelihood is that more of these treatments will become available in the future.

Given that very extensive clinical trials have shown that these drugs can be highly effective in reducing the chances of cancer coming back, it is rather surprising that surveys have shown that people often don't actually take them. For example, a recent study from Ireland discovered that within a year one in five women will have stopped their tamoxifen, and by three and a half years more than a third will have given up on the drug. These figures were based on actual prescription records and so probably give a more accurate picture than other surveys, which largely relied on asking the patients themselves. It seems an obvious message, but if your doctor has given you medication that they think will reduce the likelihood of further problems from your cancer, then do make sure you take it regularly, as prescribed.

Screening

It is also important to remember to carry on taking part in routine cancer screening. The three national screening programmes in the UK are for cervical cancer and breast cancer in women, and for bowel cancer in everyone over the age of 60. Sometimes people think that if they have had one type of cancer they cannot get another, and so they do not need to carry on with regular screening tests. This is not the case; having had breast cancer successfully treated sadly doesn't mean you can't get cervical cancer or cancer of the bowel at some time in the future. Likewise, having had a cancer of the colon or rectum, or a cancer of the cervix doesn't always protect you against breast cancer.

In the same way, having had a normal screening test for one type of cancer doesn't mean that there cannot be a different cancer in another part of your body. Each test is specific and only looks for one sort of cancer. For example, having a normal mammogram is reassurance that you are very unlikely to have breast cancer, but the test only looks at your breasts and cannot detect cancer anywhere else. Many people do not realize that this is the case, and I have often had women attending my breast cancer clinic who have been amazed that they have been diagnosed with the condition because they recently had a cervical smear test that was reported as normal, and they thought that this meant they could not get cancer.

So, you should carry on taking up the invitations for your regular screening check ups when they are due, in order to maximize your protection against further problems.

6

Everyday life after cancer: sex and fertility

There is such a thing as normal life after cancer, but finding your way back into it can often be difficult. In the next four chapters we will look at important aspects of everyday living that can be changed by a diagnosis of cancer, and its treatment, exploring some of the problems and offering some advice on how to cope.

Sex and relationships

The diagnosis of cancer and the treatment that follows that diagnosis often have a huge effect on people's sex lives. Unfortunately, for many this effect will be negative. In 2008 the charities Cancerbackup and Relate published the results of a survey of 372 people affected by cancer; 215 of those who responded had had cancer themselves, and the remaining 157 were partners of people with cancer. Overall, nearly nine out of ten (86 per cent) of the respondents said that cancer had put a strain on their relationship, and more than two-thirds (72 per cent) said that cancer had affected their sexual relationship.

These changes may be due to a shift in your emotions, so that for one reason or another you just don't feel like sex, or it may have a more physical cause, such as severe tiredness, difficulty in getting an erection or vaginal dryness and discomfort.

A change in your emotions

One important point to make clear at the start is that having sex does not increase the risk of your cancer coming back. Many people feel too shy or embarrassed to ask their doctors and nurses about this, and so often worry unnecessarily that making love could cause a relapse. There is absolutely no medical evidence that this is ever true, and you need have no anxieties or inhibitions on this score. If this is all that is holding you back, then forget the misconceptions and take up where you left off before you were diagnosed.

Although there is no medical reason why you should not continue your normal love life after your cancer treatment, many people won't find this reassurance enough and will still have very mixed or uncertain emotions about the thought of sex. The first and most important step in handling this change in your feelings is talking, and the most important person to talk to is your partner. Many people find that talking about sex, and in particular their own needs and emotions, is not easy, but letting your partner know what you are experiencing is essential, so that you both can reach a shared understanding of the way you are feeling. Talking may be hard but it is far better than hiding your worries and concerns, or trying to pretend that things are normal when they are not.

Every relationship between two people is different, and each has a different mix of things that hold that relationship together. However, love, mutual respect, and a desire to protect and care for your partner are common cores to most couples that can be drawn upon. These should be the background that makes talking about difficult subjects a positive way forward for both of you, whereas secrecy and uncertainty can be much more damaging.

Usually, partners will be understanding, supportive and sympathetic. Once you break the ice and bring up the subject of sex, finding ways forward together to adapt to your altered desires and emotions should become easier, and you will at least have created a starting point from where you can work together to sort out any problems that your change in sexuality is causing in your relationship.

For some couples communication is more difficult, and even just starting to talk together about anything as sensitive as sex may be hard. If this is the case then counselling may be a help. A trained counsellor might well be able to overcome the reservations, inhibitions or anxieties that are holding back an open discussion of the subject, and not only help sort out what the problems are but pave the way to find solutions to those problems. Quite a few hospitals do have counsellors available for their cancer patients, and there are also sources of help outside the National Health Service (NHS). Once this background awareness of the situation has been established, you can go on to look at ways of coping with it.

The most likely difficulty is a mismatch in desire, with the person who is having treatment feeling less sexy whereas their partner's libido remains much the same. This is very natural for both parties, and neither of you should be guilty about the way you are feeling. Once again, talking helps in reaching an understanding that your physical desires are different, and that that difference is entirely reasonable. From that basis of acceptance of difference, you can begin to sort out how to handle the situation. The solutions will be different for different people. They might include an agreed abstinence or a period of celibacy till you both feel the time is right; alternatively, you might adjust your relationship to one of hugs, caresses and cuddles, showing your love physically without actual sex, or you might change your approach to sex, with a greater emphasis on things like touching, stroking and masturbation, rather than penetrative sex, or changes in position that make actual intercourse more relaxed and less tiring.

These adjustments can only be made by you both, and can only be achieved by talking and understanding. There are no rights and wrongs, no set rules, for how the sexual dynamics of a couple should change at these times. So finding out what works for you is the right answer, rather than thinking there is some magic formula that you ought to try and follow.

Depression and anxiety

Sometimes emotions do get out of control and the most likely focus for this is an increase in anxiety or depression. Being worried about whether your cancer might come back, or fretting over side effects of treatment and when and whether they will get better, is entirely natural and understandable. Sometimes, however, these worries can take over your life and dominate your feelings, so that you can rarely relax or put them out of your mind. It is possible that these stresses may tip you over into clinical depression. This leaves you feeling constantly low and sad, lacking the will or energy to do anything, often sleeping badly and losing interest in everything, including food and sex. A loss of sex drive is almost always part of the picture of clinical depression. If you feel that worry or depression, with constant anxiousness or hopelessness, are taking over your life then do get help. Talk to your family doctor, or your oncologist or your specialist nurses; anxiety and depression can often be very easily treated. It may mean some sessions of counselling, or taking some simple drug treatment for a few weeks, but the results can be dramatic and transform your life back toward normality. These are not problems that you should suffer, when such easy, safe and effective help is available.

Some physical issues

There are some practical, physical issues that are also worth mentioning.

After radiotherapy to the pelvis or after some types of chem-otherapy and hormone treatments, many women will find that they have vaginal soreness and dryness that can make intercourse uncomfortable or even painful. Sometimes this can be due to fungal infection in the vagina, caused by reduced immunity caused by your treatment. In this case the soreness is often accompanied by itching and irritation, and sometimes a white or yellowish vaginal discharge. If this happens then a short course of antifungal drugs will usually clear this up very quickly, in a matter of a few days. So if you suspect that you have this problem, then do mention it to your nurses or doctors.

After radiotherapy to the pelvis there is sometimes a risk of some inflammation of the vagina that may lead to scar tissue forming (doctors call this fibrosis). This fibrosis may make your vagina narrower and more rigid, making intercourse uncomfortable or even painful. At most hospitals where radiotherapy is given, there should be a specialist nurse or radiographer who will see you before and during your treatment to warn you about this possible side effect. They will usually give you a dilator and lubricant that you can use regularly to help stop scar tissue forming. It is important to follow their advice and, in particular, to continue using the dilator and lubricants after your treatment is over, because it is during the 12 or 18 months after radiotherapy that the fibrosis begins to form, not during the treatment itself. You therefore need to carry on with them, and to keep in touch with your specialist nurse or radiographer so that they can continue to advise you.

Vaginal dryness often develops because of hormonal changes caused by your treatment (these may only be temporary and disappear a few months after treatment is over, but they can still be unpleasant at the time). If vaginal dryness is a problem, then there are a number of solutions. There are a variety of lubricants that you can buy at chemists or supermarkets that you and your partner can use; these include KY jelly, Senselle, Sylk and Astroglide, or simple glycerine can be used as an alternative, although unlike the others it is not water soluble and so is a bit more sticky. Another alternative is Replens, which again can be bought over the counter. This is a moisturizer that comes as soft white gel packaged in special applicators for easy vaginal insertion.

There are also creams or gels for vaginal use which you can only get on prescription. These contain small amounts of the female hormone oestrogen, which nourishes the lining of the vagina and makes it more moist. These include Vagifem, Ovestin, Premarin and Ortho-Gynest (these may not always be suitable for some women who have had breast cancer). So, if vaginal discomfort is a problem and over the counter treatments haven't helped, do talk to your medical team about it; there may be a very quick and simple solution.

Problems with getting an erection

Men may often find that getting an erection is more difficult after radiotherapy to the pelvis, pelvic surgery or some types of hormonal and chemotherapy. If there is a physical basis for the difficulty, as a result of either the treatment given or the effects of the cancer itself, then drugs like sildenafil (Viagra), vardenafil (Levitra) and tadalafil (Cialis) may help. These are only available on prescription, so you would need to discuss this with your doctor. Other solutions for physical problems include small injections of drugs like papavarine or alprostadil (Caverjet, Viridal), which you can be taught to give as injections directly into the penis, or – in the case of alprostadil – as pellets inserted to the penis. Another approach is the use of vacuum pumps, which can be attached to the penis before intercourse, to stimulate an erection. Sorting out the right approach to this problem can be difficult and it is something where you probably need to talk to your doctor to get his or her advice on what can be done to help.

Change in quality of orgasm

Sometimes radiotherapy to the pelvis, or some types of chemotherapy, can lead to a reduction in the amount of semen that a man produces. This means that when you ejaculate you may notice that only a small amount of fluid is produced from the end of your penis. For some men, it may mean that no semen at all is produced, resulting in what is known as a *dry ejaculation.*

Other men find that although they are still able to have an orgasm, the sensation feels different from before. Sometimes the sensation may feel less intense, or it may take longer to reach orgasm. This may be due to changes in the blood flow in your pelvis as a result of treatment or it may be the result of psychological changes. If the difference in sensation is a problem, then having a word with your family doctor and asking whether you can see a specialist sex counsellor may help.

In the same way, women who have had a hysterectomy as part of their treatment, pelvic radiotherapy, or some types of hormone therapy may find that although they can usually still achieve an orgasm, it may feel different from how it used to be. Once again, if the difference in sensation is a worry then having a word with your family doctor or your specialist nurse might be worthwhile.

Hormone replacement therapy for men

Very occasionally, cancer or its treatment can lead to a lack of male hormone: testosterone. This is most likely for men who have had testicular cancer who have had to have both of their testicles removed as part of their treatment (the testicles are the main source of testosterone in the body), or who have had radiotherapy or surgery to certain areas of their brain that might have damaged their pituitary gland (which produces hormones that stimulate the production of testosterone by the testicles). Along with problems with getting an erection and a loss of interest in sex, a low level of male testosterone is also likely to lead to tiredness, loss of energy, mood changes and baldness. Blood tests will be able to confirm whether there is a deficiency of the hormone, and if these show that there is a problem then HRT is possible. This usually involves wearing skin patches containing testosterone, but sometimes skin gels or long-acting injections may be used as an alternative.

Changes in your appearance

Another physical factor that may influence your sex life is a change in your physical appearance, or body image. This may be due to treatment you have had, such as an operation like a mastectomy, where a breast has been removed, or bowel surgery that has left you with a colostomy. Alternatively, it may be that you have either lost or gained weight during your treatment, or had other cosmetic changes, such as altered hair colour and texture after chemotherapy.

Once again changes in body image affect everyone differently. Some people take them in their stride and feel that a change in their physical appearance has little or nothing to do with the real 'them' and makes no difference to the person they really are. At the other extreme, some people feel completely devastated by the change and suffer a huge loss of confidence. Likewise, the effect on partners can be very variable, with some feeling that a mere physical change has not altered the person they know and love, whereas others find the altered appearance more unsettling. It is also the case that what you feel may be very different from what your partner feels. The survey mentioned at the beginning of this chapter found that among people who had had cancer, almost three out of four (74 per cent) found they lost confidence and felt less attractive because of their cancer diagnosis and its treatment. In contrast, among the partners questioned, only one in five thought that the experience had changed how attractive their partner was to them.

Talking is the key to adjusting to this situation. The likelihood is that if you have concerns then your partner is going to be less affected than you are. They will therefore be able to offer you reassurance that 'you' are still the person they love and care for, and that any change in your appearance makes no difference to those feelings.

In terms of physical sexuality, you or your partner might at first find that change off-putting. The probability is that after talking about it that feeling would lessen or disappear. However, if it remains a cause of tension, then it might be possible to get round it by adjusting the technique of your love making so that you could hide the change, covering the area with a sheet, say, or keeping certain bits of clothing on during intercourse. Sometimes these new ways of love making actually lead not only to a renewal of desire but also to increased enjoyment with the novelty of the new approaches to sex.

Fertility

Fertility, the ability to father a child or to become pregnant, can be affected by both cancer and its treatment. Reduced fertility directly due to the cancer itself is relatively uncommon, but treatment can quite often have an effect.

If surgery includes the removal of both a woman's ovaries, or her womb, or both a man's testicles, then sterility is inevitable (if only one ovary or testicle is removed then fertility may be slightly reduced but it is still quite possible to become pregnant or father a child).

Radiotherapy is only likely to cause infertility if the ovaries or the testicles are directly included in the area that is being irradiated. For example, if a woman has radiotherapy to her pelvis, then it is very likely that her ovaries will be affected, whereas if she is having radiotherapy to one of her breasts then there is no risk that her ovaries will be damaged. Total body radiotherapy, which is used to treat some leukaemias and lymphomas, will generally lead to infertility because the ovaries or testicles will be included in the treatment. Both the ovaries and the testicles are very sensitive to radiation, and if they are damaged by the treatment this injury is usually permanent. Radiotherapy can also affect a woman's womb, and if this organ has received anything other than a relatively low dose of radiation then it is very unlikely that a pregnancy will be possible.

With chemotherapy the picture is more mixed. Some chemotherapy drugs are very likely to cause permanent sterility, damaging both the ovaries and the testicles, whereas others may simply reduce fertility for a period of months after treatment, and yet others have no effect at all on the patient's ability to have children. This situation is complicated by the fact that with many of the newer chemotherapy drugs the long-term effect they have on fertility is still uncertain. One other consequence of some types of chemotherapy is that the drugs will lead to a premature menopause, with the ovaries stopping production of the female hormones some years earlier than might have been expected. The likelihood of this happening is, unfortunately, very difficult to predict.

The main hormone therapies that suppress ovarian or testicular function, such as the drug Zoladex, all have a reversible effect. While you are having the drug your ovaries or testicles will not be producing the hormones necessary for conception, but once you stop the treatment normal hormone levels should return within a few months, and fertility will usually return to its pretreatment level.

Testing for fertility after treatment

If surgery has involved removal of a woman's womb or both her ovaries, then sterility is unavoidable. After radiotherapy and chemotherapy the situation is less certain. With certain drugs and higher doses of radiation, the ovaries are very likely to be permanently affected, but with other drugs or lower doses of radiation the outcome is less predictable. As well as the treatment itself, the woman's age is a factor, in that the younger she is the less likely it is that her ovaries will be permanently affected.

Chemotherapy and radiotherapy affect a woman's ovaries in two ways. They cause damage to the female eggs stored in the ovary, and they also damage the cells that make the female hormones: oestrogen and progesterone. Sometimes the eggs may be more affected than the hormone cells, and this may mean that although her periods come back after the end of treatment, a woman may still be infertile. If infertility is a possibility then the usual way to test for this is to take blood samples to measure the hormone levels. Because these change over time it may be necessary to carry on testing for as long as 6 months before doctors can be sure that a woman has become infertile.

For men, radiotherapy and some types of chemotherapy will damage the male sperm in the testicles, but will have little or no effect on the hormone producing cells, so male sex hormone levels are not usually affected by these treatments, and infertility is purely the result of damage to the sperm. This means that infertility testing for men is done by sperm counts. These look at the number and quality of the sperm in samples of semen produced by masturbation. The time it takes for sperm production to recover after treatment varies considerably; sometimes it may be only a matter of a few months, but it can take as long as five years, and after certain types of treatment it will never recover.

Pre-treatment precautions

Although this book is aimed at people who have completed their cancer treatment, describing what can be done to help before treatment starts will explain some of the points that are mentioned in the next section.

It is certainly true that in the past oncologists didn't always mention the risk of infertility to their patients before they started treatment. Studies have suggested that in up to half the cases in which there might have been a risk, this was not discussed. In some cases, this might have been because they simply did not think of it, giving all of their attention to the need to treat the cancer and give the best chance of a cure. In others, it might have been because the need to start treatment was so great that there was no time for discussions about the risk that it might lead to sterility. In recent years, however, much more attention has been paid to this particular problem, and it should always be explained before treatment starts.

If their treatment carries a risk of permanent infertility, then men should usually be offered the chance of sperm banking. In the UK this is available for men of any age, and their sperm is usually stored for up to ten years. Normally two sperm samples are taken, about a week apart. These are obtained by masturbation, and the semen is then frozen and stored. All cancer centres should have counselling and sperm banking services available, and these are usually (but not always) free of charge on the National Health Service. Although the service is widely (and usually freely) available, statistics show that only about three out of ten men who are offered sperm banking actually use it.

The options for women are much more limited. Unfortunately, the female eggs, unlike the male sperm, are very easily damaged by freezing, and so 'egg banking' is not routinely possible. However, this is an area where a lot of research is being done, and this may make it more widely available in the future. A similar approach is the storage of a sample of tissue taken from the ovary by means of an operation. This is then frozen and re-implanted in the pelvis after the end of treatment. This is also an experimental treatment and is not routinely available, but it may become more widely used if results prove successful. The most widely used approach at the moment is embryo storage;

fertilized embryos will survive freezing without any damage. This involves collecting female eggs and fertilizing them, in the laboratory, with sperm from the patient's partner to produce the embryos. These are then frozen and then re-implanted into the woman's womb after the end of treatment. However, this takes some time to arrange, because it may need a period of hormonal treatment before the eggs are collected. Therefore, it may not always be possible, because it could dangerously delay starting treatment for the cancer.

Help available to couples where one partner is infertile after cancer treatment

Infertility resulting from cancer treatment can lead to much increased emotional distress. Not surprisingly, research has shown that people wanting to have children after cancer treatment who find that they are infertile, or have had their fertility reduced, suffer problems with unresolved grief, depression, anxiety and generally reduced satisfaction with life. It often colours their whole existence. Unfortunately, the problem may often be insoluble, but there are a number of ways in which the medical team may be able to offer some help.

Fertilization after sperm storage

If a man has been rendered sterile by his treatment, and he preserved some of his sperm by sperm banking before treatment, then artificial insemination of his sperm is a service offered by the National Health Service. This involves injecting some of the stored sperm into his partner's womb at the time she is ovulating. Although artificial insemination is widely available, many fertility clinics are replacing it by more sophisticated *in vitro* fertilization (IVF) methods, which may help to increase the chances of achieving a successful pregnancy.

Donor insemination

A different approach that may be considered by women whose husband/partner has been sterilized by treatment and who does not have stored sperm available is donor insemination. This means that sperm is provided by donors (who are approved and registered with the Human Fertilisation and Embryology Authority). Donors are usually matched to provide as close a fit as possible to the couple's physical and racial make up. The donor's sperm is then inseminated into the female partner's womb.

A similar technique, using eggs or embryos from female donors, which have been fertilized by sperm from their partner and which can then be implanted in their womb, is sometimes available to women who have been sterilized by cancer treatment. This may be suitable for some women made sterile by chemotherapy treatment because, although treatment may have permanently stopped her ovaries from working, it usually will not have had any effect on her womb. This is in contrast to pelvic radiotherapy, in which the irradiation of the womb may make a successful donor pregnancy more difficult, with an increased risk of miscarriage or a premature birth.

Partly as a result of new legislation that came into effect during 2006, which gives the resulting child the right to have information about their parents (including names and contact details) once he or she is 18 years old, there has been a considerable fall in the number of donors available.

Donor insemination is a complex emotional and ethical decision, and couples who are considering it will always need to go through a period of professional counselling to help them.

Surrogacy

Surrogacy is a completely different way of solving the problem of infertility. This is where another woman carries a baby for an infertile couple. Although it is legal in the UK, this option is only very infrequently used.

Adoption

This is an option, and people cured of cancer will still be considered by adoption agencies, but at present there are relatively few children available for adoption in the UK, and waiting lists are likely to be long.

Having children after cancer treatment

Even if you have no problems with fertility after your cancer treatment, the thought of having children can still raise many questions. Three of the most common worries are as follows.

- Will treatment have an effect on any future children?
- (For women) Will becoming pregnant increase the risk of my cancer coming back?
- Will treatment increase the chance of problems during my pregnancy?

Will treatment have an effect on any future children?

The main concern here is around chemotherapy, and whether the drugs used cause genetic damage to a woman's eggs, or a man's sperm, which might mean that if they parent children at a later date, those damaged eggs or sperm might lead to birth defects or other health problems in those children. Happily, there is absolutely no evidence that this is the case. Studies have looked at the children born to people after chemotherapy and have found no increase in the number of health problems. So, if you have had chemotherapy and want to parent children, then this is one worry that you do not need to have.

If asked, doctors will often recommend that you don't become pregnant, or father a child, for about six to twelve months after finishing chemotherapy. This is to make sure that any final traces of the drugs are out of your system and that things are back to normal. The actual scientific evidence for this advice is really very minimal and it is usually given 'just to be on the safe side', rather than being based on any studies showing that there might be a risk to future children if you go ahead sooner.

Will becoming pregnant increase the risk of my cancer coming back?

The general answer to this is 'no'. Most research on the subject has been done looking at women who have had breast cancer, and the results show no evidence at all that becoming pregnant after treatment is over increases the chances of breast cancer coming back. Indeed, there is at least one study that shows the risk is actually slightly reduced. The results from other cancers show a similar picture, with no suggestion that becoming pregnant will cause a relapse. As always, there may be certain individual circumstances that make an exception to this principle, so if you are thinking of becoming pregnant it is always a good idea to chat this through with your oncologist and obtain their advice.

In the past, doctors have tended to make a recommendation that a woman shouldn't get pregnant until two years after her cancer treatment is finished. Although there are various reasons for this, the main one is that most relapses occur in the first two years after treatment, and if you have a relapse when you are pregnant this could make treatment much more difficult, and possibly less successful. There are also the more social anxieties about having a new born baby when your life expectancy might have been dramatically reduced by the return of the cancer. However, set against these considerations is the growing awareness that women who have had cancer treatment, and chemotherapy in particular, are more likely to have an early menopause – even though they may have retained or recovered their fertility – and so have a reduced window of opportunity to become pregnant. This has led to suggestions that the 'two year rule' might be reduced to a delay of only six months. This is very much an individual decision, weighing up the different factors involved and how important they are to you personally. Once again, it is always advisable to seek your oncologist's view, so that you can have some expert advice to guide you.

Will my treatment increase the chance of problems during my pregnancy?

The answer to this depends on exactly what treatment you have had in the past. In many instances there will be no risk of increased problems, but this is not always the case. For example, if you have had a course of radiotherapy to your pelvis, which has involved a relatively high dose of radiation to your womb, this might increase the chances of having a miscarriage or giving birth prematurely. Also, certain types of chemotherapy may lead to some complications. For example, a number of chemotherapy drugs cause minor damage to the muscle of the heart. Usually, this is not a problem and is not something that you are likely to notice, but pregnancy puts considerable strain on the heart and might lead to symptoms of breathlessness and fluid retention, or mild heart failure. Any possible complications that might occur during pregnancy as a result of previous treatment can usually be predicted and then managed and treated, so that the pregnancy is successful and relatively trouble free. The key to this, however, is forward planning by an expert medical team. Yet again, if you are planning a pregnancy, talk to your doctors and seek their advice.

A final word

If all of this sounds very daunting, do take comfort. Many young people who have had cancer go on to be parents of healthy, happy children. Research looking at those families show they often feel that the previous illness has enriched their experience and makes them better parents, believing that their past experience helps them cope better with daily stresses and traumas, and leads them to place greater value on family closeness.

7

Everyday life after cancer: work

Each year in the UK almost 100,000 people of working age will be told that they have cancer. Some may be able to carry on working during their treatment, whereas others may have to reduce their working hours or have some periods of time off. Others still may have to give up work completely for weeks or months. What happens, though, when your treatment is over? To a great extent this depends on your age and attitude. If you are older and close to retirement, then it may be an easy decision to give up your job, but if you are younger you may have more of a dilemma. There is also the fact that our feelings about work vary from person to person. For some of us the job we know, with its routine, its pleasures and the company of friends and colleagues, is the focal point of our lives, and giving up would be unthinkable. In contrast, for others it is a treadmill of drudgery and boredom that they can't wait to leave behind. Of course, there is also the financial aspect of work. A generous pension may make retirement an easy choice, but if giving up your job, or even reducing your hours, might mean real difficulty in making ends meet and carrying on the lifestyle you enjoy, then decisions become much harder and you may have to make difficult choices.

Research has shown that two other factors that influence whether people go back to work after their cancer are the treatment that they have had and the amount of sick leave they have taken. A recent British survey by Macmillan Cancer Support found that of those people who had surgery as the only treatment for their cancer, nine out of ten returned to work. Among

those who had received either radiotherapy and/or chemotherapy or hormone therapy, only seven out of ten went back
to work, and they generally took longer to go back than those
who had received surgery alone. Perhaps unsurprisingly, the
same survey also found that of those people who took less than
12 months off work to cover the period of their treatment and
recovery, nine out of ten went back to work, but of those who
took more than a year's sick leave only six out of ten returned
to work and one in ten stopped work altogether.

What many people do not realize is that you do have 'rights'
in this situation. As someone with cancer, you are covered by
the Disability Discrimination Act (DDA), and this applies even
after your treatment is over and you have been given the 'all
clear'. Interestingly, a survey conducted in 2006 showed that
although most employers did know that the DDA applied to
people who had been treated for cancer, a worrying 20% (one in
five) did not. It is therefore worth having a look at what the Act
says, so that you have some idea of what your entitlements are.

The Disability Discrimination Act

The DDA was introduced in 1995 and modified in 2005. Some
of the changes in 2005 were relevant to people with cancer, and
these included the statement that they would be '... deemed
to be covered by the DDA effectively from the point of diagnosis, rather than from the point when the condition has some
adverse effect on their ability to carry out day-to-day activities.'
So once you have been told you have cancer, you are then
protected by the DDA, whether you are still having treatment
or not, and whether you have any health problems from your
cancer or not.

The 2005 amendments to the Act go on to say that for
people with cancer, or a history of the disease, '... it will be
unlawful for an employer to discriminate against job applicants

or employees' and '... employers will have to consider what reasonable changes to their employment conditions, recruitment policies and procedures they may need to make for people who they know, or could reasonably be expected to know, have cancer'.

The DDA covers virtually all aspects of the employment process, protecting people who have had cancer from discrimination in the following areas.

- Recruitment: an employer must not refuse to consider you for a job simply because you have had cancer.
- Terms and conditions of employment: your employer should not change the nature and requirements of your job without your agreement.
- Opportunities for promotion: you should have equal rights with your colleagues when it comes to chances of improving your position.
- Training and benefits: you should have the same opportunities as your fellow workers for going on courses and getting any perks that are offered by your employer.
- Unfair dismissal: your rights are protected.
- Unfair treatment compared with other workers: you should not be singled out for different treatment from your colleagues simply because of your history of cancer.
- Harassment and victimization: from either your immediate managers or fellow workers.
- Employment benefits: you should continue to receive the same benefits as before your cancer, including health insurance, holiday allowances, opportunities for overtime and so on.

The DDA also states that if someone has some degree of disability or their health is still impaired after their cancer treatment, then their employer must make 'reasonable adjustments' to their workplace and working practices to make sure that people with a degree of disability are not at a significant disadvantage compared with their colleagues. What these 'reasonable adjustments' actually are will vary from individual to individual, and whether the changes that need to be made can be considered 'reasonable' or not will depend on factors such as the cost of making the changes, the amount of difference those changes will make to the employee, how easy it is to make those changes, and whether they will affect the employer's business or other workers. If some of these issues are a problem, then a scheme that may be able to help is the Government's 'Access to Work' programme.

Access to work

The Access to Work scheme is organized by the Department for Work and Pensions, and is operated through Jobcentre Plus. It is for people who have a disability or health condition that is making it difficult for them to get back to work, and this includes people who might have health problems as a result of their previous cancer or that is caused by side effects of treatment. The scheme offers financial help and might meet some of the costs of the equipment you need at work, of adapting the workplace to meet your needs or of employment of a support worker to help you. It can also pay toward the cost of getting to work if you can't use public transport.

You may be able to get support from Access to Work if you already had a paid job or if you are unemployed and about to start a new job; it can also help people who are self-employed. If you have a disability or health problem after your cancer that stops you from being able to do parts of your job or may have a long-term effect on how well you can do your job, and this is likely to last for 12 months or more, then this scheme may be for you.

If you wish to explore whether Access to Work might help you, the first step is to ask the Disability Employment Adviser at your local Jobcentre Plus office about Access to Work. They will then put you in touch with your closest Access to Work Business Centre to check whether you're eligible for help. If you are eligible, you will be given an Access to Work adviser, who will then speak to you and your employer to find out what your needs are, and how best they can be met.

Once your adviser has worked out what support they feel you need, they will apply for approval of this from Jobcentre Plus. You and your employer will then receive a letter telling you what support has been approved and what funding is on offer to help with this. It is then up to your employer (or you if you are self-employed) to make the necessary arrangements in the workplace, and they (or you) can then claim back the contribution to the costs of this that was agreed by Access to Work. The actual amount of that grant will have been agreed previously between your employer and your Access to Work Adviser, but – depending on your circumstances – it can be anything from 80 to 100 per cent of the costs involved. Any financial help you receive is for a maximum period of three years, after which the Access to Work Business Centre will review your circumstances and the support that you are receiving.

When to go back to work

Surveys suggest that, generally speaking, medical advice about going back to work has tended to be fairly unhelpful. Unless your doctors feel that there is a particular problem with your fitness, which might mean that you should not return to your job, then their guidance has usually been along the lines of 'no reason why not, it's up to you, when you feel ready', with possible suggestions that you 'take it easy to begin with' or 'feel your way back in gently, don't overdo things'. However, even though their advice may be limited to 'yes' or 'no', it is still important to check with your doctors that they are happy for you to return to work, and that they do not foresee any health related problems.

To be fair to your medical team, there are aspects of your health and wellbeing that only you can really know for sure. These include how tired you feel, how much energy you have and how much you can do mentally and physically without feeling worn out. Neither will your medical team have detailed knowledge of what your job involves, the demands it makes on you and what it means to you. This latter point is something that often changes after a diagnosis of cancer and a period of treatment, and this change can go in any of several directions. Returning to work may be an important part of your journey back to complete recovery, returning to normal and putting your cancer behind you. Alternatively, you may find that life's priorities have altered and that you want to spend more time with family and friends, or pursuing interests and hobbies rather than going back to your full time job. You may also just feel that it is time for a new direction in your employment and to look for a new job – a new beginning for a new you. You may feel like looking for a new job because you want a challenge, a stimulus to reinvigorate your life, or it may be that – having been away from it for some time – your old occupation seems too dull, too busy or no longer suits you for some other reason. Then again, or you may feel that things have changed while you've been away and that it will be difficult to fit in with new routines and catch up with changes in your previous workplace.

Although your family and friends may all have opinions, someone else who may be able to offer valuable advice about your return to work is your employer. Most larger companies will have an occupational health officer, and talking to them should be very helpful because they have the knowledge and experience to guide you through weighing up the pros and cons of returning, and they may also be able to suggest ways to make your return to work easier and more likely to be successful and long lasting. Ask your manager or human resources team whether there is an occupational health expert who you can see. If your company doesn't have one you could go privately to an independent adviser, and your employer might even pay for this if you ask them. Alternatively, if you belong to a trade union or professional organization, they may be able to help.

Going back to work

The specific person within an organization who handles your return to work and how it is managed will vary, but one factor that plays a major role in your return is the size of the organization. Some large companies may have a formal policy already in place for managing employees who have had cancer, but they are in the minority; others will have a 'chronic illnesses' policy that they can adapt to meet the particular needs of people who have had cancer, but many will have no guidelines in place to handle your situation. If this is the case, then there are two documents produced by national charities that your managers might find helpful. These are 'Working through cancer: a guide for managers' (produced by Macmillan Cancer Support, and available on their website: <www.macmillan.org.uk/work>) and 'Cancer & working: guidelines for employers, HR and line managers' (produced by Cancerbackup in collaboration with employers organizations and available online: <www.cancerbackup.org.uk>). Obviously, you can look at these as well and you may find them helpful.

The first step in planning your return to work is to set up a meeting with your employer to give you both the opportunity to explore fully your needs and options. Some companies may offer an employee assistance programme with confidential counselling and advice, so do check whether this is available, although unfortunately it is the exception rather than the rule.

Your return to work interview is likely to be with your manager, someone from the human resources department, or possibly someone from the occupational health team. This is an important meeting and you may find it useful to have someone with you to help you remember everything that is said, and to make sure that you get all the information and support you need. This might be a family member, a friend, a work colleague or a union representative.

Everyone's needs will be different in this situation, but the following list gives some ideas of things you may want to achieve during your return-to-work interview.

- Work out a timetable for coming back to work, which might be a step-wise pattern, gradually building up your hours over a period of time; agree a schedule for this.
- Decide whether you need to or want to alter your working pattern on a longer term basis, possibly going part time or working more flexibly or with some element of home working.
- Confirm your entitlements to breaks and holidays.
- See whether this gives you the opportunity for an agreed change in your role and responsibilities.
- Check whether you need any retraining or to go on any refresher courses to catch up with changes that might have taken place while you were away.
- Possibly arrange for some informal visits to get the feel of things again before you actually start back at work.
- Let your employers know if there are any changes needed in your workplace to meet any special needs that you may have after your cancer treatment.
- See whether you need help with transport to work, or special parking arrangements, or whether you need to adjust your hours to avoid rush hour travel.

Once you have an agreed plan for your return to work, it is

a good idea to arrange with your employer another meeting a while after you have started back, so that you can check that everything is going to plan and that you are coping with things.

Financial consequences

Returning to work will almost certainly alter your financial position. Often, it will mean more money coming in as you get back into paid employment, but sometimes there can be a negative effect as well, losing entitlement to some benefits that you may have been receiving during your time on treatment. These issues are covered more fully in the following chapter.

8

Everyday life after cancer: money matters

Being told that you have cancer opens the floodgates to all kinds of anxieties and problems. To begin with, these will almost certainly focus on your long-term outlook and treatment. For instance, can your cancer be cured, and what will you have to go through in terms of surgery, radiotherapy or chemotherapy in order to win through, and what side effects might you have to face along the way? However, once the emotional turmoil of the initial diagnosis and treatment begins to settle, as your life adjusts to your dramatically changed circumstances other worries can begin to surface, and for many people these include difficulties with money. In 2004 a survey by Macmillan Cancer Support suggested that more than three out of four people in the UK diagnosed with cancer suffered some financial hardship, and in 2008 the same charity estimated that of the 1.2 million people in Britain living with the consequences of cancer some 400,000 were likely to need guidance in managing their finances and making ends meet. Indeed, for many people worries about how they would cope financially caused them more stress than their cancer and its treatment.

There is much help on offer for people with cancer, but the evidence is that this help is often not taken up. One estimate suggests that every year more than £126 million in state benefits are not claimed by cancer patients who are entitled to them. For some this may be a matter of pride, not wanting to feel that they are dependant on Government hand outs (even though these belong to the person with cancer by right – a right that they have often paid for in life-long taxes and national insurance contributions). For others it is often the case that they simply do not realize what is available to them.

Everyone's circumstances and needs will be different, and the range of support that is on offer is constantly changing. Also – and especially when it comes to state benefits – the range of options, who qualifies for them and what you actually get can be very confusing. This chapter can only provide a general picture, but I hope that it will serve as a first step along the road to helping to sort out any money worries that you may have. To do this the chapter is subdivided into four areas: who you can turn to for advice; some thoughts on managing your personal finances; the state benefits that are available; and some of the other agencies that might be able to help.

Who can help you?

Your family and friends may be able to offer some useful advice and helpful tips, but there are many other sources of help. If you are still having regular check ups at hospital then the medical team is well worth talking to. It is unlikely that your oncologist will have all the necessary information at their fingertips, although your specialist nurse may have a good idea of what options are open to you. It is most likely, however, that they will arrange for you to see either a hospital social worker or a Macmillan nurse working at the hospital, who will have more detailed knowledge of what is on offer. Alternatively, they may arrange an appointment with the local Patient Advice and Liaison Services. From 2007 onward the National Health Service is introducing 'information prescriptions' for cancer patients. These should include a range of leaflets, booklets and other sources of information tailored to meet the needs of individual patients, and should provide some financial guidance. However, the availability of these information prescriptions is rather patchy, and their quality is variable.

If you are not attending hospital, then your general practitioner may well be able to put you in touch with your local Macmillan nurse, or may have a social worker based at the health care centre who might be able to give you some guidance.

The Citizen's Advice Bureau is staffed by people who can provide good advice, and they are very experienced and knowledgeable when it comes to the confusing maze of state benefits. They also have staff who can provide guidance on legal issues. Their advice is free and their contact details should be in the telephone directory, or you can look at their website: <www.citizensadvice.org.uk>.

A number of the national cancer charities have leaflets or booklets on financial problems, and Macmillan Cancer Support is particularly active in this area. They have a free booklet called 'Helping with the cost of cancer', which you can obtain by ringing their free hotline (0800 500 800) or visiting <www.macmillan.org.uk/abetterdeal>. This is part of their 'Better Deal' campaign to help ease financial hardship among people who have had cancer. This campaign recently (April 2008) got a boost with generous financial support from the Royal Bank of Scotland, and the plan is to use the new funds to extend the provision of welfare and financial advisers as well as to finance a benefits helpline providing advice on such matters as housing and council tax benefits, and help with prescription costs. All being well, these should be in place by the time this book is published.

A number of Government agencies can offer help. Your local Jobcentre Plus can give advice about claiming benefits (the address will be in the phone book or on <www.jobcentreplus.gov.uk>). The Department for Work and Pensions has a range of leaflets on benefits; these are often available at local post offices and libraries, but they can also be downloaded from their website: <www.dwp.gov.uk/resourcecentre>. There is also the national freephone Benefit Enquiry Line (0800 882 200) for people who are ill or disabled, including those who have had cancer.

If debt is a problem or likely to be an issue, then The National Debt Line offers free advice, which is completely confidential. They can be contacted on 0808 808 4000 or at <www.nationaldebtline.co.uk>.

If you are thinking of returning or have returned to work, then your employer may be able to help with advice from the human resources team. If you belong to a Trade Union, there may be staff who can provide specialist advice. Another alternative is to contact an independent financial adviser. They can look in depth at your situation and needs and make recommendations, although this usually involves some form of payment. You can find out about independent financial advisers in your area at the Find a Professional website: <www.findapro.co.uk>.

Finally, if you have a local Cancer Support Group in your neighbourhood, they may well have lists of useful contact addresses, and leaflets or booklets on handling financial problems.

Managing your personal finances

It may be that you have been lucky and that your cancer and its treatment have had very little impact on your day to day life, and now all that is behind you and you are able to carry on much as before. However, if your circumstances have changed, and your income has been affected, then you may need to look at some aspects of the way you manage your money. This might include reviewing insurance, retirement and pensions, mortgages and loans, among other factors, and you may need to consider the possibility of obtaining outside help with grants.

If you have insurance policies that relate to your general health and fitness, it is worth looking at what they cover and checking with your insurance company whether you are entitled to make a claim. The type of policies that might be relevant include income protection, critical illness cover and some private medical insurance schemes. If you have private medical insurance as part of your employment package, then it is possible that there might be some benefits that you can claim from this, and your manager or your company's human resources team might be able to advise you.

If you were working before your cancer was discovered but you now have doubts about returning, you could explore the possibility of early retirement. This would normally mean taking a reduced pension from your previous employer, but if you have any long-term disability as a result of your cancer or caused by a side effect of your treatment, then it might well be possible to retire on medical grounds, which will often considerably increase the amount you are entitled to. One possible positive result of having had cancer when it comes to retirement is that many companies will give increased annuity payments to people who have had treatment in the past. Annuities can be quite complicated and people often don't realise that they can choose between different providers. Cancer Research UK has recently started a new service for people who have had cancer and want to find out more about their annuity choices. This can be accessed on the Cancer Research web site by looking under the Cancer Research UK Retirement Service or calling them on 0845 094 1905. Once again, if you are thinking about early retirement, check with your employer or their HR team, or your Trades Union representative to see what might be on offer.

For most of us our mortgage is the major financial burden that we have to carry, representing the main drain on our monthly income. If mortgage repayments are a problem, check whether you have any insurance policies linked to your mortgage that might give you some protection and cover some of the costs. If not, then it may be possible to agree a lower monthly rate of repayment by remortgaging at a lower rate, or extending the period of your borrowing, especially if you have already paid off some of the capital on your property (so that you have equity in your property). Alternatively, you may be able to change to a loan based on interest payments only for a period of time. The key thing here is to let your lender know about your change in circumstances and to talk to them about the options that are available to you.

On a similar theme, look at all your regular outgoings – payments that are made weekly, monthly or once a year – and check whether any of these can be stopped or reduced. For example, subscriptions to organizations you are no longer interested in, insurance policies that are no longer necessary or charitable donations you can no longer afford. If you are facing a short-term problem in your finances, then it is sometimes possible to agree deferred payments of things such as rent, council tax and energy bills, giving you a few months to sort your income out. Talk to your landlord, local council and energy supplier to find out whether they offer such a scheme. Likewise, if you have outstanding loans on credit cards or store cards, check whether these can be swapped to companies charging lower interest rates or whether you can negotiate a lower rate of monthly repayments.

Sometimes, it may be possible to get one-off payments or grants to cover a particular money problem or to meet a particular bill. If you belong to a trade union or another professional organization, they may have a benevolent fund that could offer help, so it is worth contacting them. Macmillan Cancer Support will also provide financial help for people who are in difficulty from the effects of their cancer. You have to apply for these with the help of a Macmillan nurse, another health care worker or the Citizen's Advice Bureau. Also, the grants are means tested, so they are not available to single people who have savings in excess of £6,000, couples with joint savings in excess of £8,000 or families with a disposable income of more than £100 per month per person.

State benefits

The benefits system is complicated and confusing, and many people simply don't make a claim because they do not realize what they are entitled to. Other people simply feel embarrassed about taking 'charity' or asking for help, but it is important to recognize that these benefits are yours by right, and if you are eligible you should not hesitate to take advantage of them.

The benefits system is changed or adjusted quite regularly; the following account gives an overview of what was available in mid-2008, but you should check to make sure things haven't changed. Some benefits are means tested and only given to people on lower incomes or with little in the way of savings, but others are more widely available. These include Statutory Sick Pay, Incapacity Benefit, Disability Living Allowance and Attendance Allowance.

Statutory Sick Pay

If you have been working and making national insurance contributions, then you should receive Statutory Sick Pay from your employer for the 28 weeks that you are off sick. (This may be a continuous period of sick leave or a number of episodes relating to the same illness.) You need to let your employer know about your illness and give them a doctor's certificate after your first week off work. Your employer will then pay you at the Statutory Sick Pay level in the same way as they paid your salary. This is a minimum payment determined by the Government, but your employment contract may guarantee a more generous allowance, so do check on this. If you are still not back at work after 28 weeks then you can claim Incapacity Benefit.

Incapacity Benefit

If you were not working when your cancer was discovered or if you are still unable to return to work after 28 weeks, then you can claim Incapacity Benefit provided that you have paid sufficient national insurance contributions and you are under the age of 65 years. This benefit is organized through Jobcentre Plus, and they will be able to find out whether you have paid enough national insurance. They will also arrange to assess your incapacity. This benefit is paid at three different rates.

- Short-term lower rate: for the first 28 weeks of illness for people who are not getting Statutory Sick Pay.
- Short-term higher rate: from 28 weeks up to one year off work.
- Long-term rate: when your incapacity lasts more than a year.

If you were not working when your cancer was discovered and you do not have enough national insurance contributions for Incapacity Benefit to be paid, then you will probably be eligible for some of the means tested benefits mentioned below in this chapter. At the time of writing, the Government has announced that in late 2008 Incapacity Benefit will be replaced with a new payment called the employment support allowance. Details of this will be available on the web site <www.direct.gov.uk/en/ DisabledPeople/FinancialSupport/esa/index.htm>. People who are already on Incapacity Benefit will continue with it as before.

Disability Living Allowance

Disability Living Allowance is for people under the age of 65 years who need help with their care, and this includes people who are left with a disability as a result of their cancer or side-effects of treatment. The allowance is determined based on the level of your disability and is not related to your national insurance contributions or any other income or savings you may have; it is also tax-free. There is a time factor in that you usually need to have had your disability for at least three months, and it is likely to continue for at least another six months. You can claim Disability Living Allowance even if you are still able to work and even if you do not have anyone to give you the care that you need (in other words, you don't have to have a carer to get the allowance). The allowance is paid at several different levels depending on your degree of disability and your needs. These are grouped under two different headings: the care component and the mobility component. If you get Disability Living Allowance under the mobility component you will also get the Blue Badge, allowing free parking in most places, and free road tax.

If you are entitled to Disability Living Allowance it is likely that your medical team will have all of the necessary information to help you to claim it, but if not you can get claim forms from your local Social Security office.

Attendance Allowance

This is broadly similar to Disability Living Allowance but is for people over the age of 65 years.

Means tested benefits

There are a wide range of benefits available to people who are on low incomes or who have little or no savings. The type of benefit and the amount you receive varies with your individual circumstances. These benefits include Income Support, Pension Credits and Jobseeker's Allowance. There also Tax Credits from the Inland Revenue (Child Tax Credit and Working Tax Credit), and benefits from your local council (Council Tax Benefit, Housing Benefit and free school meals) and grants for children over 16 years who are continuing in full time education. You may also be eligible for help with medical costs, including free prescriptions and payments for travel costs to hospital.

Having so many different benefits and allowances makes finding out just what is available and just what you are entitled to quite a daunting task. The Citizen's Advice Bureau are very good at helping you through the maze of benefit options, or you could contact your local Social Security office or ring the Benefit Enquiry Line (0800 882 200).

Incidentally, if you have been claiming benefits and then decide to go back to work this can affect your entitlements. Disability Living Allowance and Attendance Allowance are both paid whether you are working or not, and if you return to work but your earnings are low then you may still be able to claim any means tested benefits. Incapacity Benefit stops if you return to work, however, although if you find you are not coping and have to give up work again you can restart the benefit, at the same rate, provided that you apply within 56 days from the time when you stopped it.

Other sources of help

As well as Macmillan Cancer Support, a number of other charities may offer one-off payments to people who have had cancer. The CLIC Sargent organization is specifically for young people affected by cancer and gives grants to people under 21 years old. Applications have to be made on your behalf by a health or social worker, but you can find out more about what might be on offer by calling (020 8752 2825) or e-mailing (<grants@ sargent.org>). The Association of Charity Officers is an organization that helps to point people in the direction of particular charities that might be able to help them financially, and they can be contacted by telephone (01707 651 777) or through their website (<www.aco.uk.net>). In addition, some charities that limit their involvement to a particular type of cancer may have funds available, and it is worth checking with your specialist cancer nurse to see whether she or he knows whether this might be an option for you.

Many local councils offer what are called Direct Payments. These are grants that can be used to pay for a variety of things, including help with personal care, short breaks away from home, help with transport costs and help to access community services. These grants are available to older people or disabled people over the age of 16 years or to carers aged 16 years and over. For more information, contact the Social Care department of your local council.

It seems an injustice, but many people who have had cancer have to pay for their prescription charges, even if the drugs are essential to prevent their cancer coming back. If you do have to pay for your prescriptions and need regular medication, a pre-payment certificate may help. These can be for either four or 12 months, and will work out cheaper if you need more than five items in four months, or 14 items in 12 months.

A final point to mention is that if you think your cancer might have been caused as a result of your job (e.g. working with asbestos or dangerous fumes or chemicals), then you may be able to claim for compensation from your employer or you may be eligible for the state payment of Industrial Injuries Benefit. The Department for Work and Pensions can give you more details about this (their website is: <www.dwp.gov.uk>).

9

Everyday life after cancer: holidays and travel

For many people one of the most important ways of celebrating the freedom brought by the end of cancer treatment is to plan a holiday. A holiday can be a way to draw a line under a period of intense anxiety and disruption, a key step along the path back to a normal life, a way to gain reassurance that you truly have recovered, or it can just be a chance to have a really great time. Regardless, the fact that you can now think about a complete break, a revitalising change of scene can often be enormously significant. There can be problems, however. Is it safe to go away, especially if you are planning a long journey to an exotic destination? What precautions, if any, do you need to take? What about taking essential medication out of the country? Can you go out in the sun? What about vaccinations and the potentially expensive issue that can still cause problems years after your treatment is over, namely travel insurance?

Is it safe to travel?

This question is likely to be most relevant in the immediate aftermath of treatment. If you have had major surgery, then it will probably be a few months before you are ready to travel any great distance. If you have had surgery on your lungs or your brain, then there may be specific restrictions about flying, and you should check with your surgeon if you are planning this. Chemotherapy can often leave you with a lowered level of immunity and increased susceptibility to infection, which can last anywhere from a few weeks to some months. Therefore, delaying a holiday – particularly if it is to a more exotic or isolated location, where infection risks may be high and medical facilities limited – may be wise. If your cancer or its treatment has left you with any tendency toward shortness of breath, anaemia or lymphoedema (swelling of an arm or leg due to problems with the lymphatic system), then flying might make symptoms worse.

Another potential problem is that many cancers lead to increased risk of developing deep vein thrombosis – the formation of blood clots, particularly in the veins of the legs. Long haul flights, which frequently involve sitting still in a relatively cramped position for considerable periods of time, also encourage the formation of deep vein thrombosis, and so people who have recently had cancer are at particularly high risk if they make these journeys. How long the increased tendency toward deep vein thrombosis lasts after successful cancer treatment is not clear, but if you do make a long haul flight then taking routine precautions to reduce the risk – getting up and walking around the plane at regular intervals, wearing elasticated support socks or stockings, and avoiding dehydration (no alcohol and lots of water) – would be a wise move. Furthermore, if you have had breast cancer and are still taking tamoxifen as part of a long-term programme to reduce your risk of the cancer coming back, then you should be aware that tamoxifen may increase your likelihood of developing a deep vein thrombosis, so you should make sure that you do take the precautions that have been recommended.

The whole experience of cancer and its treatment, especially if you have had radiotherapy or chemotherapy, can also leave you profoundly tired for some time afterward. That tiredness may last for weeks, or even months, and may often be a level of fatigue that makes even the routine chores of everyday living a considerable burden. In these circumstances you may well feel that a holiday is just too much of an effort, and it is important not to be persuaded by well meaning friends and relatives to take a break until you feel that you have energy to enjoy it and make the most of it.

This brief section just gives you an idea of some of the things to bear in mind if you are thinking of a holiday after the end of your treatment, but everyone's circumstances are different. To get advice and guidance that is best suited to your needs, it is a very good idea to have a chat with your oncologist or your specialist cancer nurse, to hear their thoughts on how safe it is for you to travel, whether there are any restrictions on what you can do or where you can go, and any precautions that you need to take.

Vaccinations

For some overseas destinations it may be necessary to have vaccinations to protect you against various infectious diseases that may be endemic in that part of the world. Occasionally, this can be a problem after cancer treatment.

Vaccines work by stimulating our immune system to produce antibodies that will remain in our blood and kill off the bacteria or viruses that cause the infection. There are two types of vaccine: live and inactivated. The live vaccines use small doses of the actual cause of the infection ('germ') to stimulate our immunity. The inactivated types use 'germs' that have been killed by heat or chemicals, or extracts from those germs; although they are effectively dead, these germs (or extracts from them) can still be recognized by our immune system and lead to antibody formation.

Some types of cancer, such as leukaemias and lymphomas, and some cancer treatments – in particular certain forms of chemotherapy – can reduce our levels of immunity, and this reduction may last for months after the treatment is complete.

If our immune system is impaired and a live vaccine given, there is the risk that our natural defences won't be strong enough to cope with it, and instead of becoming immune we could actually develop that infection and become quite ill. Alternatively, if an inactivated vaccine is given, and our immune system is not working properly, then although we won't get the infection (because the vaccine is 'dead') it might mean that we won't be able to produce the antibodies in response to the vaccine. It will therefore be ineffective, and we won't be protected against the infection.

The main infections for which a live vaccine is required for protection are as follows: measles, mumps, yellow fever, and polio and typhoid (oral vaccines of these two). The important infections for which an inactivated vaccine is used are as follows: diphtheria, tetanus, hepatitis A and B viruses, rabies, and polio and typhoid (injectable vaccines for these two). The advice is that if you are planning a trip to a part of the world where vaccinations are recommended, check with your medical team to find out about your level of immunity and whether it is safe for you to have these vaccinations, and whether they will give you effective protection.

Going out in the sun

After treatment for a cancer, especially if that treatment involved either radiotherapy or chemotherapy, people are frequently uncertain about the dangers of going out in the sun. Specifically, they may be concerned about whether they are more likely to get sunburn or whether sunlight might increase the chances of their cancer coming back.

As far as the chances of cancer coming back are concerned, going out in the sun will have little effect one way or the other; there is no good evidence that sunbathing makes a recurrence of cancer more or less likely. However, there is the general warning that too much sunshine increases our likelihood of getting skin cancer. On the other hand, a lot of our supply of vitamin D is produced by our skin when it is exposed to sunlight, and that vitamin D is essential to keeping up our levels of calcium (which we need for healthy bones). So, people who remain permanently out of the sun are likely to have lower levels of vitamin D, lower calcium levels and an increased risk of bone disease. (Also, recent research has suggested that an increased risk of breast cancer might also in some cases be linked to low levels of sunlight.) So, what is the right balance? The UK Health Department and Cancer Research UK have issued excellent advice in their Sun SMART campaign. The key messages are as follows.

- Avoid going out in the sun between 11 a.m. and 3 p.m., or if you do go out keep in the shade.
- Make sure you never burn. Sunburn isn't just painful – it doubles your risk of skin cancer.
- If you are going out in strong sunlight, cover up with a t-shirt, hat and sunglasses. When the sun is at its peak sunscreen isn't enough.
- Children should be especially careful; young skin is delicate, and getting sunburn as a child is even more dangerous than getting it in later life.
- Use a sunscreen of sun protection factor (SPF) 15 or greater and apply it generously; remember to reapply it often.

So, like many other things, sunlight is fine – in moderation.

If you have had radiotherapy, then for at least a year after treatment the skin that has been irradiated will be more sensitive than normal to sunlight, so if you are out in the sun, and your treated skin is going to be exposed, use a sunblock of at least SPF 15 to protect against sunburn. This increased tendency toward sunburn only affects the skin that has actually been affected by your radiotherapy treatment; other areas do not change in their response to sunlight, so if the radiation was given to a part of your body that you would normally keep covered then there really isn't a problem.

The effects of chemotherapy on the skin are variable. Some of the drugs used will make your skin more sensitive to sunlight, and more likely to burn. This change may last for many months, or even years, after your treatment is over. Other drugs have little or no effect. In general, hormone based treatments won't alter your sensitivity to sunlight. Your medical team may be able to give you specific guidance as to whether your treatment might have made your skin more sensitive, but if you are unsure then start with fairly short times in the sun, using a sunblock, and if that is OK and causes no problems then you can gradually increase your exposure.

Taking medication on holiday

Although your cancer treatment is over, you may still need long-term medication, taking tablets to help control side effects of past treatment, or as part of a long-term programme to reduce the risk of your cancer coming back. There are a few things to bear in mind about your drugs, particularly if you are going abroad. The most obvious of these is to make sure you take enough with you; it is wise to take extra to allow for any delays on your travels, and to take enough to let you temporarily increase the dose if this might be necessary (e.g. with some painkillers or long-term steroids, such as prednisolone). Usually, your GP will be able to prescribe any additional tablets or medicines that you need, although the maximum supply they can give is usually three months. Therefore, if you plan to stay abroad for longer than this, you may have to explore how to get further supplies while you are still out of the country. Do keep a note of your drugs, their strengths and doses with you, so that if they should get mislaid you can try to obtain replacements. Incidentally, always use the generic, or scientific, name of the drug itself, not the brand name or trade name, because these can vary from country to country. A final tip is to suggest that you take some of your medication in your hand luggage and pack some in your cases, so that if your bags do get separated or lost at any time, you still have a supply of your medication with you.

The situation is more complicated when it comes to controlled drugs. These are drugs covered by the Misuse of Drugs Act, and – for people who have had cancer – the most likely ones to be relevant are strong pain killers, such as morphine, which may occasionally be necessary to help ease painful after effects of the cancer or its treatment. The Government changed its regulations on the personal transport of these drugs in January 2008. If you are going abroad for less than three months, you can take all the controlled drugs you need for your trip, but you must have a covering letter from your family doctor. This letter must include your name, address, date of birth, your dates of outward and return travel, the country(s) you are visiting, and the names, doses and total amounts of the drugs that you are taking with you. If you are staying abroad for more than three months then you will need to apply for a special licence from the Home Office. If you are travelling with a controlled drug(s), you should keep it in your hand luggage, and make sure it is in its original packaging with the labelling giving details of doses and quantities; also, you will need your doctor's letter to show to customs officials. A final point is that the country or countries you are visiting may have restrictions on the controlled drugs you can bring into them. This may affect the amount of the drug you can transport or it may be a difference in the way they are classed; for example, some countries count codeine as a controlled drug, so it may be wise to check with the British consulate of the country you are planning to visit to check on their regulations. The Home Office website gives details of contact numbers for these consulates and full details on taking these drugs overseas (<www.drugs.homeoffice.gov.uk/drug-laws/ licensing/personal>).

Getting insurance cover

Obtaining insurance cover is often one of the biggest head-aches for people who have had cancer and then want to go on holiday. Sometimes, long after their treatment is over and fol-lowing years of good health, people still find that mentioning a past history of cancer can cause real problems in obtaining travel insurance. In 2005 a survey by Macmillan Cancer Support found that four out of ten people who had had cancer ran into difficulties when they tried to obtain holiday cover, and one in 20 had cover refused completely.

The trouble is that insurers view a history of cancer as a 'pre-existing condition' – something that might still be present and could lead to a need for further medical treatment, which might be very costly. As a result, they may do one of a number of things: they might refuse to insure you; they might charge you a higher than normal premium (and there are lots of horror stories of huge sums of hundreds or even thousands of pounds being asked); they might charge you an excess (so that you have to pay the first £50, £100 or whatever sum they name, of any medical charges); they might impose special conditions (such as not covering any expenses related to cancer treatment); or they just might offer you a normal policy. What happens is – to a considerable extent – a lottery, depending on which insurer you contact, and the all important message is to shop around to look for the best deal, because there are enormous variations on what is on offer.

When you do contact an insurer it is important to mention your previous cancer, because if anything does happen, and it is realized that you concealed this information, then your policy will be invalid and you will have to bear all of the costs yourself.

Insurers will vary in how they handle enquiries from people who have had cancer; some will have a blanket policy, others will take account of your individual details to try and personalize a quote for you. This will often involve a telephone interview with a specialist nurse or other expert. These interviews can be quite upsetting because they may bring back painful memories of distressing treatment and stir up old anxieties, but the insurers do have to get as accurate a picture as possible to work out the risks involved in taking you on as a client. The fact that insurers can raise questions, and create doubts about whether a past cancer has been cured, can also make you wonder whether what your doctors have told you was true. If they told you that you were almost certainly cured but the insurance company says that you are still at risk, who is right? The answer to this is that your doctor is correct because they know you and your past medical history much better than any insurer ever can. In fact, some insurers may ask for a letter from your doctor, to back up what you tell them, before they will give out a policy (your doctor will always do this, but they may make a small charge for the service).

The difficulty in obtaining insurance may depend on your destination. Going to the USA, where medical fees are very high, can often be a problem, whereas with European countries things are often much easier. This is helped by the European Health Insurance Card (EHIC). The EHIC has replaced the previous E111 form, which is no longer valid. Having the EHIC means you can get free or reduced cost emergency treatment within the European Union. In some cases you may still have to pay for your treatment but can then claim back the money later. The EHIC does not cover continuation of routine treatment that you are having in the UK; neither will it meet the expenses of getting you back to Britain in an emergency.

You can apply for an EHIC by post, with a form available from your post office, or by telephoning (0845 606 2030) or going online (<www.dh.gov.uk/travellers>). Applying online is quickest, and you will normally get your card in about a week; if you apply by post it could take about 3 weeks. On their website (<www.dh.gov.uk/en/PolicyandGuidance/ Healthadvicefortravellers>) and in their leaflet 'Health Advice for Travellers' (available from most post offices or GP surgeries), the Department of Health provides more detailed information. This includes a list of the countries covered by the EHIC and a number of other locations that have some reciprocal agreements with the UK for providing emergency health care. Although the EHIC does offer some cover, the official advice from the Government is that you should always obtain personal travel insurance as well.

I said it above, but it is an important message and bears repeating – if you have had cancer and are looking for travel insurance, do shop around and contact a number of companies. Their willingness to insure you, the premiums they will charge and the conditions they will impose will vary tremendously. A number of insurers do specialize in helping people who have had cancer. The details of these companies are constantly changing, so rather than give a list here I suggest that you get in touch with one of the major cancer charities such as Cancerbackup, Macmillan Cancer Support, Cancer Help UK or Breast Cancer Care, all of which have regularly updated lists of contact addresses available. (The contact details for all of these organizations are provided in the next chapter.)

10

Support for cancer survivors

Until recently the National Health Service (NHS) had largely overlooked the needs of patients once their cancer has been treated. The focus has always been on trying to improve the outcomes of that treatment – increasing the chances of cure. During the past 50 years the results of this effort have been very considerable, and great improvements have been made in cure rates of many types of cancer; in my professional life time I have seen conditions such as Hodgkin's lymphoma and secondary testicular cancer change from being universally fatal to almost always curable. Likewise, in breast cancer the long-term survival rate has moved from less than 50 per cent to 80 per cent, and it is still increasing. It is probably true to say that in general the medical opinion has tended to be that if your cancer has been successfully treated, then all your problems are over; you've survived a life-threatening illness and can now enjoy the years ahead. The fact that surviving cancer is not without its problems is a penny that has been slow to drop among health professionals.

That situation is changing. In 2007 the Government's Cancer Reform Strategy document had a whole section devoted to the issue of 'Cancer survivorship' and outlined a new 'National Cancer Survivorship Initiative', which the Department of Health would take forward in partnership with Macmillan Cancer Support and other cancer charities. The intention is to consider a range of approaches to survivorship care and to explore how these can best be tailored to meet individual needs. The agenda includes looking at the following:

- how clinical follow up should be done;
- patient education, with self care and expert patient programmes;
- provision of drop in centres for peer support;
- making more use of telephones for health professionals to keep in touch with patients and *vice versa*;
- the provision of rehabilitation programmes;
- offering psychological and spiritual support;
- more support for people who want to go back to work;
- access to financial and benefits advice; and
- guidance on diet and nutrition.

There are also plans to look in greater detail at people's needs and preferences for care at the end of treatment and what role they wish to take in managing their own care – in other words, finding out what the patient wants.

The first step in realizing these ambitions was a think tank event, 'Making the cancer survivorship agenda a reality', which was held in March 2008. At the time of writing (June 2008), a report of that event has appeared. The full text of the document is available on the Macmillan Cancer Support website (www. macmillan.org.uk/Documents/Support_Material/Get_involved/ Campaigns/Survivorship/survivorship_report.pdf). Essentially, it describes the range of issues that were discussed and the ideas that were put forward. Leading on from this there will now be an initiative, led by the Department of Health, to try to develop these concepts into practical improvements in the support and care on offer to people who survive cancer. This is to be welcomed but it will take time, and it is likely to be some years before major changes are seen. So where can people turn to in the meantime?

Cancer support groups

Another source of both support and information can be a local cancer support group. These give the opportunity for people who have, or have had, cancer (and their relatives and carers) to meet on a regular basis and talk together about their experiences. Discovering that other people have had similar thoughts and fears to yours can often be very comforting, realizing that the issues you are facing are not something you have to confront alone, and can share with others, and sometimes learn from their experience.

The idea of cancer support groups developed informally during the 1980s and they have grown in number since that time. There is no fixed pattern, and so they vary from place to place. Sometimes, they are run by specialist nurses from the hospital (in which case they often focus on one particular type of cancer), or they may be based in the community, either associated with a local health care centre, a church or a community centre. What the various groups do have in common is the opportunity to meet other people who are in a similar situation to you, or who have been through the same sort of experience in the past, so that you can compare and contrast perspectives in a social setting. There is often some form of professional input, with informal talks from experts in various fields on one or other aspect of the subject, and there is likely to be a supply of suitable background information, or someone who can give advice on where to get such information. There may also be other activities, such as complementary therapies or access to spiritual support from local faith leaders.

If you are interested in finding out more, your specialist nurse at the hospital should have details of local cancer support groups, or they may be listed in the telephone directory. Alternatively, Macmillan Cancer Support gives help to more than 800 groups across the UK and the details of these are on their website (<www.macmillan.org.uk>).

Complementary therapies

Many people turn to complementary therapies to help them cope with the burden of their cancer and its treatment with conventional therapies such as surgery, radiotherapy and chemotherapy. They are not intended to cure the cancer but are used to ease any side effects of treatment and improve general wellbeing. These supportive benefits may continue into life after cancer, offering relaxation and a sense of wellbeing that enhances the quality of life.

As a doctor of conventional medicine, I would have to say that there is no evidence to suggest these therapies increase the chance of a cure, and that any therapist who claims this is the case should be treated with scepticism and caution.

It is important to understand the difference between complementary and alternative therapies. Alternative therapies are unconventional treatments given to try and actually control cancer or prevent it from coming back. Alternative therapies are often recommended with claims for activity and benefit that sound convincing but have no medical proof. Sometimes, they have actually been shown to be ineffective or even harmful, but are still being promoted to unsuspecting members of the public. They frequently involve considerable expense and insist on demanding changes in lifestyle, with outlandish diets or special supplements of 'essential elements', 'vital vitamins' or 'immunity boosting drugs', none of which have ever been scientifically proven to work. This contrasts with complementary therapies, which are safe, well understood, can actually be pleasant to have and usually have a positive effect on wellbeing. The main types of complementary therapies are the touch therapies (aromatherapy, massage therapy, reflexology and acupuncture), fitness and movement therapies (yoga, Tai Chi and Qigong), psychological therapies and diet.

Aromatherapy involves the use of essential oils. These are

plant extracts that have distinctive smells. Each of the different essential oils is believed to have particular physical or psychological effects; for example, lavender and eucalyptus help ease stress, whereas camomile reduces inflammation. The oils may be used in massage or given as inhalations or aromatic baths, or they may be applied as creams or lotions. Reflexology is based on the belief that areas on the feet match different parts of the body, and by applying pressure to these areas energy paths are triggered that can produce beneficial effects. So, it is a type of foot massage. Acupuncture is based on ancient Chinese medicine, which believes that the body's energy, or chi, moves in pathways, or meridians, beneath the skin, and by inserting needles into these meridians a healing response can be stimulated.

The fitness and movement therapies do involve more active participation, rather than just lying back and enjoying the therapy, but many people do find that they can help to ease anxiety and depression, as well as giving a bit of gentle exercise to keep up overall fitness.

The psychological therapies can be as simple as just relaxing in a quiet room listening to restful music, or they might involve working with a counsellor who teaches you relaxation techniques, or uses visualization (picturing your body and how it is working to stop your cancer coming back, or reduce the side effects of treatment). Art therapy and music therapy, using drawing or painting to channel your emotions or listening to (and sometimes taking part in) live music performances, are other approaches to psychological therapy. Many people find that these techniques can help to ease stress and anxiety and make them feel better.

Dietary changes may involve simply taking one or more supplements to your normal diet, or a complete change in the way you eat. This is one area in which the boundaries between complementary and alternative therapies do sometimes become blurred. There are many people who claim that particular diets or supplements will actually prevent the cancer from coming back. Very often, these claims are based on the belief that the change in diet will boost the immune system. Unfortunately, there is virtually no evidence for any of these claims. Also, occasionally these diets can be quite extreme and unpleasant (or expensive), and they can actually reduce your quality of life rather than enhance it. Having a normal balanced range of foods, with plenty of fresh fruit and vegetables, is very hard to beat.

Each of us is different, and people vary greatly in their responses to complementary therapies; some will feel real benefit whereas others won't notice any difference. If you find that you enjoy it and feel better for it, then that's great, but if it doesn't help then don't hesitate to stop. Sometimes, particularly with diets, people start on a new regimen and find that they really don't like it but feel they must continue or they will get worse. This is not what complementary therapies are about. They are there to improve your quality of life, not reduce it, and if you do try a new diet or any other type of complementary therapy and find that you feel more miserable as a result, then do stop it at once.

Times are changing, and many doctors of conventional medicine are becoming more sympathetic toward complementary therapies, and some cancer centres will offer these as part of their service to NHS patients. Unfortunately, however, the availability of these services in hospitals or at GP surgeries is still very patchy and variable, and it is likely that if you do want to pursue any of these options then you will have to make your own arrangements and pay for them.

The cancer charities

There is an ever increasing number of cancer related charitable organizations in the UK, working outside or in partnership with the NHS, and funded mainly by donations from the public. To list them all, and give details of their activities and contact addresses would almost require the writing of a separate directory. I have therefore chosen a selection that I think might be particularly helpful to people after the end of their treatment. I have divided these into two groups: first, charities that cover many or all types of cancer; and second, those that focus on one of the 'big four' cancers – breast, lung, bowel and prostate cancer. The websites and literature of Cancerbackup and Macmillan Cancer Support do have details of many of the organizations I have omitted, including those devoted to less common cancers.

Charities covering a broad range of cancer types

Cancerbackup is a comprehensive information service for patients. It offers a telephone helpline staffed by specially trained cancer nurses, who can provide advice on all aspects of cancer, including living with the consequences of the condition and its treatment. It also produces nearly 70 booklets and more than 200 factsheets on all aspects of cancer, including many aspects of day to day life after cancer. There are also more than 1,000 questions and answers about cancer on its website (the website also has the texts of all of the booklets and factsheets, and links to many other useful organizations). Recently, the website has added the 'What now?' section, in which people can share their experiences of life after cancer, and it also provides an opportunity to add your own story and comments. Early in 2008, Cancerbackup and Macmillan Cancer Support merged, but for the present the two organizations are retaining their separate identities and the websites, and the contact details remain different. The address for Cancerbackup is 3 Bath Place, Rivington Street, London ECA 3JR, UK (telephone [free]: 0808 800 1234; website: <www.cancerbackup.org>).

Macmillan Cancer Support is probably best known for the nursing care it offers to people with cancer, but this organization also provides a number of publications on life after cancer, with useful booklets on benefits and financial help for cancer patients, returning to work after cancer, and holidays and travel (all listed on their website). The website also has useful information on various aspects of cancer, including a directory of local cancer support groups and patients' stories about cancer. The charity can also offer financial help, with special grants to some people who have had cancer. The address for Macmillan Cancer Support is 89 Albert Embankment, London SE1 7UQ, UK (telephone [free]: 0808 808 2020; website: <www.macmillan.org.uk>).

DIPEX is a charity that offers a website for people to share their health related stories. The initials stand for 'Database of individual patient experiences'. The site covers a number of different illnesses but has an extensive section on cancer. This not only provides some background information on various types of cancer but also many stories from people who have had cancer, giving you an opportunity to learn from their experiences and to add your own comments. The website is at the following address: <www.dipex.org>.

Cancer Research UK is mainly known for the work it does to develop and test new treatments for cancer, but their website (<www.cancerhelp.org.uk>) includes a wealth of information on many aspects of cancer, including some advice on coping with the side effects of treatment, and life after cancer. Other contact details are as follows: PO Box 123, Lincolns Inn Fields, London WC2A 3PX, UK (telephone: 020 7121 6699).

Charities covering the 'big four' cancers

There are many different charities related to breast cancer, but Breast Cancer Care places particular emphasis on offering support to people (men as well as women) who have or have had breast cancer. The organization's free helpline (0808 800 600) provides further medical information, emotional support or simply more details about what the charity has to offer. There is also a website that allows you to send enquiries to the specialist nursing team, or visit forums or live chat sessions to share your views with other people who might be in a similar situation. There are also a variety of publications that you can download from the site (<www.breastcancercare.org.uk>). A special feature is that the charity has regular free two day workshops around the country specifically for people who have had breast cancer and are now looking to get back to normal life afterward.

For people who have had lung cancer, The Roy Castle Lung Cancer Patient Network offers a free telephone helpline giving access to specialist nurses, and regular monthly group meetings at which patients and their families can find out more about issues related to lung cancer. There is also a lung cancer patient involvement programme in which people who have had the cancer can help to shape lung cancer services and raise the profile of lung cancer globally. The contact details are as follows: 220 London Road, Liverpool L3 9TA, UK (website: <www.roycastle.org>).

Two charities that offer services to people with bowel cancer are Bowel Cancer UK and Beating Bowel Cancer. Both provide a wealth of written information and access to specialist nurses who can provide information and support. Contact details for the nurses at Bowel Cancer UK are as follows: telephone (free) 0800 840 3540 and e-mail <advisory@bowelcanceruk.org.uk>. Beating Bowel Cancer can be contacted on 020 8892 1331 on Mondays, Wednesdays and Thursdays from 9.30 a.m. to 1.30 p.m.; the e-mail address is <nurse@beatingbowelcancer.org>. Bowel Cancer

UK also has a patient to patient support or 'buddy' system, where people who had bowel cancer can volunteer to help others who are going through treatment, as well as providing information on living with bowel cancer. Beating Bowel Cancer also has a patient to patient support group, which aims to match people in similar situations so they can talk to one another on the phone. Further contact details for Bowel Cancer UK are as follows: 7 Reckett Street, London SW6 1RU, UK (telephone: 020 7381 9711). Those for Beating Bowel Cancer are as follows: 39 Crown Road, Twickenham, Middlesex TW1 3EJ, UK (telephone: 020 8892 5256).

The Prostate Cancer Support Association (PCSA) offers support and information for men who have had prostate cancer. It offers written information and has a national helpline (0845 6010766; e-mail: helpline@prostatecancersupport.info). The charity also runs a number of local support groups, although at the moment these are based mainly in the South East of England. The contact address for PCSA is as follows: BM Box 9434, London WC1N 3XX, UK.

Index